PSYCHOLOGY OF EMOTIONS, MOTIVATIONS AND ACTIONS

PSYCHOLOGY OF NEUROTICISM

PSYCHOLOGY OF EMOTIONS, MOTIVATIONS AND ACTIONS

Additional books in this series can be found on Nova's website under the Series tab.

Additional E-books in this series can be found on Nova's website under the E-book tab.

PSYCHOLOGY OF EMOTIONS, MOTIVATIONS AND ACTIONS

PSYCHOLOGY OF NEUROTICISM

KRISTEL PARN
EDITOR

New York

For permission to use material from this book please contact us:
Telephone 631-231-7269; Fax 631-231-8175
Web Site: http://www.novapublishers.com

Library of Congress Cataloging-in-Publication Data

ISBN: 978-1-62808-150-3

Published by Nova Science Publishers, Inc. † New York

CONTENTS

PREFACE

In this book, the authors present current research in the study of the psychology of neuroticism. Topics discussed include the measurement, development and behavioral expressions of neuroticism in early childhood; the relationship between perceived parenting styles and neuroticism in Argentinean children and adolescents; and evaluating mindfulness as a mediator of neuroticism and resilience.

Chapter 1 - Neuroticism is a broad dimension of personality characterized by proneness to negative emotionality, irritability, moodiness and vulnerability. These characteristics were traditionally studied in children by means of a temperamental dimension of negative affectivity. More recently, it has been demonstrated that temperament and personality traits share more commonalities than differences and that broad personality dimensions, resembling the Big Five in adults (including neuroticism), can be retrieved from caregiver ratings of children at least from the age of three years onwards. This contribution provides an overview of the conceptualization, measurement and development of neuroticism over early childhood, and its links to important developmental outcomes. The authors' summary of the extant research advocates that child neuroticism (and its specific trait constituents) as observed by different informants, using diverse measures of child personality and referring to target samples in several countries can be reliably rated over early childhood. Ratings of child neuroticism further show consistent concurrent and longitudinal associations with internalizing behavior and difficulties in social relationships across multiple settings, and may also protect against development of externalizing problems. Longitudinal studies of broad personality dimensions over childhood are scarce due to a fairly recent conceptualization and interest in empirical investigation of this specific field of development of individual differences. Therefore, the authors draw on their own empirical work based on questionnaire data by multiple informants and present an overview of several types of developmental and cross-informant consistency in neuroticism and its specific trait constituents. In general, adult ratings of neuroticism in young children retain a considerable mean-level consistency and show substantial rank-order stability from ages 3 to 6 years, whereas a reliable individual-level change is observed in a minority of children, with similar proportions of children increasing and decreasing in the trait. The children are consistently perceived lower in neuroticism traits by their parents than teachers. Mothers and fathers strongly agree in ratings of their child's neuroticism traits and parent–teacher agreement appears moderate. Surprisingly, boys are perceived by the adults somewhat higher in neuroticism traits than girls. Adding to the studies in the field, the authors' research also suggests that neuroticism shapes early sibling relationships, difficulties in socially competent behavior and predicts developmental trajectories of internalizing behavior across early childhood. The findings derived from a cross-lagged design further indicate that children's dispositional tendencies towards neuroticism are more likely to influence subsequent internalizing behavior than vice versa. The continuity of early childhood neuroticism as observed by significant adults, its developmental significance and possible modifications of its behavioral expressions are discussed from the perspective of person–environment transactions. Potential accounts of several other child characteristics and environmental influences on early neuroticism are also highlighted as child personality, although it shows a substantial consistency, is not set like a plaster and could be changed as well.

Chapter 2 - The objectives of this chapter are: 1). To study differences, according to gender and age, in the perception of the father and mother parental styles (acceptance, pathological control and extreme autonomy) in childhood and adolescence; 2). To study differences in neuroticism dimensions (self-criticism, vulnerability, anxiety, perceived lack of competence), according to gender and age; 3). To study the relationship of parental styles as perceived by children with neuroticism according to gender and ages. The total sample consisted of 1494 Argentinean children and adolescents. It included 517 middle-class children aged 8-11 (M = 10.26, SD = .88), both genders (253 boys and 264 girls), and 977 adolescents aged 12-16 (M = 12.85, SD = .86) both genders (431 boys and 546 girls), from primary and high schools in Buenos Aires and Tucumán, Argentina. The results indicate that father and mother parental style are perceived in a different way by children, according to gender and ages. On the other hand, the results of this study revealed statistically significant differences in neuroticism dimensions, with female children showing higher levels of neuroticism, especially self-criticism, vulnerability and perceived lack of competence, the results shown that children who show demonstrate higher levels of self-criticism, vulnerability and anxiety than adolescents. Lastly, the authors found that the only parenting dimension that is associated with neuroticism is pathological control, that is, excessive, intrusive control, based on guilt, which implies the implementation of strict norms, punishments and scolding, based on a negative evaluation of the child and distancing through rejection.

Chapter 3 - Neuroticism is implicated in negative affect predictions, and functions as a complex dimension of personality, a vulnerability factor for psychopathology, and as the primary underlying factor in trait negative affect. The research literature's consensual acceptance of neuroticism as a factor in psychological distress is well documented through research studies and meta-analyses. Neuroticism is linked to deficiencies in emotional and cognitive functioning, resulting in problems with self-regulation, attention and awareness. Neuroticism has demonstrated inverse correlations with resilience: the perceived ability to cope effectively with adverse situations (Labbé et al., 2011, 2012). Ongoing research continues to explore psychosocial variables that can effectively mitigate neuroticism's negative effects. Mindfulness, as a psychological construct and intervention based on a core spiritual practice of Buddhism, has gained acceptance in recent years due to its positive effects on a variety of psychological stressors (Baer, 2006), and its potential as an effective mediator of neuroticism (Feltman et al., 2009; Fetterman et al., 2010; Labbé et al., 2011, 2012). The cognitive qualities and emotional outcomes of mindfulness may produce mediation effects on the ineffective attention and awareness that leads to negative reactivity in neuroticism, and provide a stronger relationship with subjective resilience. Findings of recent research regarding neuroticism, mindfulness, and resilience are presented in a discussion of a mindfulness model to mitigate the effects of neuroticism on resilience. Future directions of research and strengths and limitations of current research are discussed.

In: Psychology of Neuroticism
Editor: Kristel Parn
ISBN: 978-1-62808-150-3

Chapter 1

NEUROTICISM IN EARLY CHILDHOOD: ITS MEASUREMENT, DEVELOPMENT, AND BEHAVIORAL EXPRESSIONS

Maja Zupančič[1] ***and Tina Kavčič***[*2]
[1]University of Ljubljana, Slovenia
[2]University of Primorska, Slovenia

ABSTRACT

Neuroticism is a broad dimension of personality characterized by proneness to negative emotionality, irritability, moodiness and vulnerability. These characteristics were traditionally studied in children by means of a temperamental dimension of negative affectivity. More recently, it has been demonstrated that temperament and personality traits share more commonalities than differences and that broad personality dimensions, resembling the Big Five in adults (including neuroticism), can be retrieved from caregiver ratings of children at least from the age of three years onwards. This contribution provides an overview of the conceptualization, measurement and development of neuroticism over early childhood, and its links to important developmental outcomes. Our summary of the extant research advocates that child neuroticism (and its specific trait constituents) as observed by different informants, using diverse measures of child personality and referring to target samples in

[*] Corresponding author: Tina Kavčič, Faculty of Education, University of Primorska, Cankarjeva 5, 6000 Ljubljana, Slovenia, e-mail: tina.kavcic@pef.upr.si OR tina234@gmail.com.

several countries can be reliably rated over early childhood. Ratings of child neuroticism further show consistent concurrent and longitudinal associations with internalizing behavior and difficulties in social relationships across multiple settings, and may also protect against development of externalizing problems. Longitudinal studies of broad personality dimensions over childhood are scarce due to a fairly recent conceptualization and interest in empirical investigation of this specific field of development of individual differences. Therefore, we draw on our own empirical work based on questionnaire data by multiple informants and present an overview of several types of developmental and cross-informant consistency in neuroticism and its specific trait constituents. In general, adult ratings of neuroticism in young children retain a considerable mean-level consistency and show substantial rank-order stability from ages 3 to 6 years, whereas a reliable individual-level change is observed in a minority of children, with similar proportions of children increasing and decreasing in the trait. The children are consistently perceived lower in neuroticism traits by their parents than teachers. Mothers and fathers strongly agree in ratings of their child's neuroticism traits and parent–teacher agreement appears moderate. Surprisingly, boys are perceived by the adults somewhat higher in neuroticism traits than girls. Adding to the studies in the field, our research also suggests that neuroticism shapes early sibling relationships, difficulties in socially competent behavior and predicts developmental trajectories of internalizing behavior across early childhood. The findings derived from a cross-lagged design further indicate that children's dispositional tendencies towards neuroticism are more likely to influence subsequent internalizing behavior than vice versa. The continuity of early childhood neuroticism as observed by significant adults, its developmental significance and possible modifications of its behavioral expressions are discussed from the perspective of person–environment transactions. Potential accounts of several other child characteristics and environmental influences on early neuroticism are also highlighted as child personality, although it shows a substantial consistency, is not set like a plaster and could be changed as well.

INTRODUCTION

Neuroticism is conceptualized as one of the broad or robust personality traits – the dimensions of individual differences in enduring tendencies to feel, think and act in a relatively consistent way over time and across contexts (e.g., Funder, 2001; McCrae & Costa, 2003). In general, neuroticism or emotional instability (vs. emotional stability) is characterized by a propensity to negative emotionality and over-reactivity to emotionally arousing stimuli at the high end and by poise, confidence, tendency to respond calmly and weakly to emotional arousal, and to recover quickly from distress at the low end. The dimension is one of the most widely used and central in almost any adult personality scheme (Angleitner, Kohnstamm, Slotboom, & Besevegis, 1998).

Many researchers have adopted the Five-Factor Model (FFM) to summarize the hierarchical organization of many narrow or specific personality traits in adults across countries and language communities (e.g., McCrae & Costa, 1997; McCrae, Terracianno et al., 2005). The model covers five broad dimensions of personality: extraversion, agreeableness, conscientiousness, neuroticism, and openness, with neuroticism or emotional instability depicting specific traits such as anxiety, worry, irritability, moodiness, vulnerability to emotional distress, wide swings in emotions, and lack of self-confidence. From the developmental perspective, the adult personality dimensions provided by the FFM have also served as targets in search for their precursors in childhood.

Until about two decades ago, child personality was predominantly conceived in terms of temperament (e.g., Ahadi & Rothbart, 1994; Buss & Plomin, 1984; Caspi & Silva, 1995; Hagekull, 1994; Thomas & Chess, 1977, 1982) – constitutionally based, early emerging individual differences in emotional, motor and attentional reactivity, and self-regulation (Rothbart & Bates, 1998; Rothbart & Derryberry, 2002). Personality traits, understood to represent social and cognitive elaborations of early temperament, were assumed to develop during middle childhood when children display an increasingly differentiated and complex range of individual differences (e.g., Caspi, 2000). Only scarce empirical studies of personality models for classifying individual differences in childhood were published before mid-nineties of the past century (Digman, 1963, 1989; Digman & Inouye, 1986; Eysenck, 1965; Eysenck & Eysenck, 1980). Factoring the questionnaire data based on adult ratings of school-age children, these studies recovered a relatively independent factor of neuroticism but in general, neuroticism was thought to be mapped onto childhood temperamental negative affectivity (Rothbart, Posner, & Hershey, 1995).

This chapter is organized around several topics concerning manifestations of neuroticism over early childhood. First, past research on developmental links of individual differences in early child temperamental negative affectivity and inhibition with neuroticism, and important developmental outcomes is reviewed briefly. Then, extant knowledge about the structure of child neuroticism is introduced, mainly from the perspective of the FFM. An outline of contemporary instruments to assess child individual differences in neuroticism is also given. Findings on several types of developmental and cross-informant consistency of neuroticism and its constituent trait-scores as obtained by adult reports over early childhood are provided in a following section. Next, concurrent and later behavioral manifestations of early childhood neuroticism are evidenced. Possible origins of continuity/change in child neuroticism and its relations to significant outcomes are addressed. The chapter concludes with accounts for limitations of the recent research on early child neuroticism and offers several suggestions for future work in this domain.

Temperament in Childhood and Developmental Links to Neuroticism

Individual differences in children, traditionally described as temperament, have been studied for over fifty years. A considerable effort has been devoted to determine the structure and developmental manifestations of early temperamental differences. Diverse temperament models have been proposed but virtually all contend that temperament has a multi-dimensional nature, includes several behavior-influencing traits and provides a foundation for later developing personality (see also De Pauw & Mervielde, 2010). The most influential models of Thomas and Chess (1977; Thomas, Chess, Birch, Hertzig, & Korn, 1963), Buss and Plomin (1984), and Rothbart and colleagues (1981; Rothbart, Ahadi, Hershey, & Fisher, 2001; Rothbart & Putnam, 2002) all comprise temperament traits of negative emotionality, which refer to a tendency to experience negative emotions, chiefly fear, anxiety, sadness, discomfort, and anger/frustration. These traits were demonstrated to be linked with neuroticism both conceptually (e.g, Caspi & Shiner, 2006; Hagekull, 1994) and empirically (e.g., De Pauw, Mervielde, & Van Leeuwen, 2009; Graziano, Jensen-Campbell, & Sullivan-Logan, 1998; Grist & McCord, 2010). The three temperament models also capture behavioral inhibition (a propensity towards shyness, fear and withdrawal from novel and/or unfamiliar stimuli), which is often related to both child neuroticism and low extraversion (e.g., Asendorpf & Van Aken, 2003; Slobodskaya, 2007) but sometimes allocated to the former (Halverson et al., 2003; Zupančič, Sočan, & Kavčič, 2009) and sometimes to the latter child personality dimension (Caspi & Shiner, 2006;

Mervielde & De Fruyt, 2002), depending on the model and/or the measure employed.

Empirical studies of Rothbart and associates (see also Rothbart & Derryberry, 2002; Rothbart & Putnam, 2002; Rothbart, 2007) explored the hierarchical structure of temperament traits in infancy, toddlerhood, early and middle childhood, and adulthood using parent and self-report (adults only) questionnaires (e.g., Rothbart et al., 2001). The factor of negative affectivity was identified across age periods. In infancy, it was defined by distress to limitations, fear, sadness, and slowly falling reactivity. Among toddlers, negative affectivity was characterized by fear, discomfort, sadness, shyness, anger/frustration, and low soothability. A very similar structure of negative affectivity was demonstrated in (pre)school children, although shyness loaded on the surgency factor, and the pattern of loadings for negative affectivity was consistent with the respective dimension found in adult data. As expected, temperamental negative affectivity in adults was related to neuroticism as measured by the FFM questionnaire.

In addition to the questionnaire data, next examples come from observation measures of early-appearing individual differences in emotional expression and temperament. The observed toddlers' emotional expressions (Izard, Dougherty, & Hembree, 1983) during episodes of the Strange Situation procedure (Ainsworth, Blehar, Waters, & Wall, 1978) showed substantial associations of sadness and anger with maternal ratings of child neuroticism (measured by Q-sort methodology proposed by John, Caspi, Robins, Moffitt, & Stouthamer-Loeber, 1994) two years later (Abe & Izard, 1999).

Remarkable evidence about continuity of early childhood temperament differences and their pervasive influences on the development in personality and social domain turned up from one of the largest longitudinal studies of human development, the Dunedin Multidisciplinary Health and Development Study (Silva & Stanton, 1996). The study (Caspi, 2000; see also Caspi, Henry, McGee, Moffitt, & Silva, 1995; Caspi & Silva, 1995) demonstrated that early-emerging temperamental differences show links to personality traits in adolescence and young adulthood, and affect life-course development in multiple contexts. One of the three large clusters of temperamental qualities that were identified from extensive observations of 3-year-olds during their involvement in cognitive and motor tasks, labeled the inhibited type, included children who were fearful, socially reticent, easily upset by unfamiliar people, and inhibited in novel situations. When the children reached age 18, they scored higher on self-described traits indexing constraint (especially harm avoidance and self-control) and lower on social potency, achievement orientation, and aggression than groups with other types of child temperament. Using a checklist of adjectives that could be grouped into five dimensions corresponding to the FFM, the same individuals (assigned to the inhibited type at age 3) were rated by others high on neuroticism and low on extraversion marker traits at age 21. The inhibited child temperament was also shown to predict later behavioral problems, mainly of internalizing nature, restricted interpersonal relationships, and low social support.

Regarding behavioral manifestations of early temperament it can be concluded that children high in negative emotionality are at risk for a variety of social difficulties as it predicts both internalizing and externalizing behaviors. However, the outcomes for anxiety and fear are often different than for irritability; the former is more frequently manifested in internalizing difficulties, whereas the latter is more predictive of externalizing behavior (Rothbart & Bates, 1998). Outcomes of shyness and inhibition similarly include low social support, high rates of anxious symptoms and other internalizing symptoms, low social competence, and poor peer-relationships (e.g., Findlay, Coplan, & Bowker, 2009). Proneness to social inhibition and different types of negative emotionality may result in similar difficulties in the social domain but for different reasons. Inhibition, fearfulness and anxiety may prevent children from engagement in their social environments, whereas irritability may alienate individuals from the social world (Shiner, 2006). In addition, higher fearfulness may predispose children toward some positive outcomes and may be considered as a protective factor against development of externalizing difficulties (see also Rothbart & Putnam, 2002; Shiner, 2006). Fearful inhibition has been identified as a form of reactive regulatory control (Rothbart & Bates, 1998) which is sensitive to punishment and early internalization of rules of conduct (e.g., Kochanska, 1997). Fearful children are thus, more guilt-prone, tend to comply more with the social rules, and behave less aggressively than their fearless peers.

Is There a Distinction Between Temperament and Personality?

Reviews of research over the past two decades have cast considerable doubts on the traditional distinction between temperament and personality, suggesting that childhood temperament traits and adult personality traits such as the FFM dimensions share more commonalities than differences (Caspi, Roberts, & Shiner, 2005; Grist & McCord, 2010; De Pauw & Mervielde, 2010; De Pauw et al., 2009; McCrae et al., 2000; Shiner, 2005). First, childhood temperament (including negative affectivity and shyness) and adult personality traits (including neuroticism) are both influenced to a similar extent by heritable genetic factors and environment. Second, many temperament and personality traits are portrayed by specific habitual valence of emotions (e.g., negative affectivity, shyness, and neuroticism are characterized by negative emotions). Third, temperament and personality involve many similar co-varying specific traits which are organized hierarchically and reveal a similar structure (e.g., specific traits such as fearfulness and sadness form both temperamental negative affectivity and personality trait of neuroticism). Fourth, personality traits of openness and agreeableness are not present in temperament models but also appear early in life, whereas some of the temperament traits (e.g., effortful control) do not emerge early after birth. Thus, the distinction between temperament and personality stems primarily from different scholarly traditions, which are increasingly converging in recent conceptualizations of child individual differences.

There is also compelling evidence indicating the usefulness of the FFM to assess individual differences among children, with neuroticism retrieved as a more or less independent factor across ages (from age 2 onwards), informants, methods of assessments, and countries (e.g., Barbaranelli, Caprara, Rabasca, & Pastorelli, 2003; Grist & McCord, 2010; Halverson et al., 2003; Knyazev, Zupančič, & Slobodskaya, 2008; Lamb, Chuang, Wessels, Broberg, & Hwang, 2002; Markey, Markey, & Tinsay, 2004; Mervielde, Buyst, & De Fruyt, 1995; Mervielde & De Fruyt, 2002).

To integrate a variety of constructs used to label child temperament or personality traits, Caspi and Shiner (2006) proposed a common taxonomy of temperament and personality traits covering individual differences emerging from early childhood onwards. The five broad dimensions in this conceptual taxonomy combines constructs from both temperament and personality frameworks, while the FFM labeling is retained. The super-ordinate dimension of neuroticism in this taxonomy integrates different aspects of emotionality, i.e. fearfulness, anxiety, sadness, and anger/irritability, whereas social inhibition is conceived as a component of extraversion. Both anger/irritability and social inhibition are thus, listed differently to the broad dimensions than it would be expected within personality traditions where the former would be, at least according to some studies, allocated to (low) agreeableness, and the latter, capturing both shyness and fear of novelty is suggested to present a combination of neuroticism and low extraversion (De Pauw & Mervielde, 2010).

Over the next sections, we will predominantly focus on portraying child neuroticism as measured within the FFM framework, particularly by adult reports on preschool children.

Conceptualization and Measurement of Neuroticism in Childhood

Consistent with the conceptual taxonomy of temperament and personality traits (Caspi & Shiner, 2006), neuroticism in the FFM studies of children is described by anxiety, fearfulness, vulnerability, moodiness, proneness to guilt, tendency towards distress, low frustration tolerance, feelings of insecurity, and lack of self-confidence. It captures propensity to experience at least three narrow traits of negative emotionality, i.e. fear, anxiety (a tendency towards general distress, apprehension, worry, tension), and sadness (low mood, dejection, hopelessness). Another two specific traits, social inhibition (discomfort and reluctance to interact with unfamiliar people and act in novel situations) and irritability (a tendency towards hostile emotions evoked by perceived limitations such as anger, jealousy, frustration, irritation) are likely to be associated with both child neuroticism and low extraversion, and low agreeableness, respectively (Shiner, 2005, 2006).

Over the past 15 years, personality traits of the FFM have been clearly identified in childhood but research has been mostly performed with adult ratings or self-ratings of school-age children (e.g., Barbaranelli et al., 2003; Digman & Shmelyov, 1997; Laidra, Pullman, & Allik, 2007; Little & Wanner, 1998; Markey et al., 2004; Van Leeuwen, Mervielde, Braet, & Bosmans, 2004). Nevertheless, a few studies evidence that a similar structure can be retrieved by adult ratings of preschool children (Asendorpf & Denissen, 2006; De Pauw et al., 2009; Grist & McCord, 2010; Knyazev et al., 2008; Lamb et al., 2002; Mervielde et al, 1995; Zupančič et al., 2009; Zupančič & Kavčič, 2004, 2009) and, using an adjusted procedure, even by self-reports of 5-year-olds (Measelle et al., 2005). Though the structure of personality traits and internal coherence of the broad dimensions over early childhood diverge somewhat from the trait structure and reliability reported from studies with older children, the dimension of neuroticism emerged across the studies with preschoolers as targets and showed a satisfactory internal consistency.

Neuroticism as Captured by the First Generation Measures of Child FFM Personality Traits

Until instruments of a new generation that are based on caregiver free descriptions of their children were constructed, variations of two approaches were employed to assess personality traits in children. Adult FFM measures with adapted item-phrasing and rating instructions to make them more suitable for child assessment were used (e.g., Markey, Markey, Ericksen, & Tinsey, 2002; Mervielde et al., 1995) or FFM scores were derived from measures that were created to operationalize another personality model, usually the California Child Q-set (CCQ; Block & Block, 1980).

Factor analyzing the scores on 100 CCQ items with different samples of Dutch children/adolescents, Van Lieshout and Haselager (1994) found a clear emotional stability factor, which summarized covariance of 16 items defined by self-esteem, self-reliance, self-confidence, calmness, relaxed behavior, tendency to recover well after stress, and by low fear, anxiety, inhibition, indecisiveness, dependence, guilt feelings, and bodily symptoms of stress. Using the same instrument with 48 items defining the FFM scales, John and associates (1994) described neuroticism as represented by two separate factors, anxious distress (anxiety, nervous worry, guilt feelings, and low self-esteem) and irritability (immature behaviors such as whining, crying, tantrums, and overly sensitive reactions). Furthermore, Asendorpf & Van Aken (2003) reported on a reliable neuroticism scale employing the short German version of the CCQ with teachers of preschool children as targets (the FFM scales were highly similar to John et al., 1994). Neuroticism was defined by fear, worry, anxiety, sensitivity to criticism, maladaptive behavior under stress and poor recovery after stress.

Various adult measures such as Costa and McCrae's NEO-FFI (see Markey et al., 2004), the M5-PreSchool version derived from Goldberg's International Personality Item Pool (see Grist & McCord, 2010) and the Flemish Big-Five Bipolar Rating Scales (see Mervielde et al., 1995) were also modified to assess the FFM traits in children. The last two examples were employed with ratings of preschool children as targets; the neuroticism scales of these assessment tools demonstrated good internal consistency, satisfactory construct validity and described emotionally instable children similarly: Worried, easily intimidated, irritable (Grist & McCord, 2010), nervous vs. quiet, tense vs. relaxed, unsteady vs. steady, and angry vs. calm (Mervielde et al., 1995).

However, all these instruments used to evaluate child personality have several limitations. The items may not represent a full range of child individual differences, since they are based on measures to assess adults and thus, some child-specific features may be obscured. Also, the items capture theorist-imposed core constructs on child personality and therefore, they may not accurately reflect those characteristics of children that are perceived salient for their parents and teachers (Knyazev et al., 2008).

Free Descriptions of Child Personality

Based on the assumption that freely generated descriptions of children by their caregivers would encode child individual differences that are salient in daily interactions, parental natural language or free-descriptive approach was adopted in a multi-national collaborative research project (Kohnstamm, Halverson, Mervielde, & Havill, 1998). Belgian, Chinese, German, Greek, Dutch, Polish, and US parents of children aged from 3 to 12 years were asked to describe their child's characteristics in their own words. In order to categorize over 50,000 statements collected, an elaborate coding system was developed, based on a combination of existing personality taxonomies and temperament models (Havill, Allen, Halverson, & Kohnstamm, 1994). The taxonomy accounts for five main FFM categories, with three subcategories each and eight additional categories. Emotional Stability represents one of the main categories and is defined by the subcategories of Emotional Reactivity, Self-Confidence, and Anxiety/Fear. The descriptions given are also coded at the high end or low end of a specific subcategory. With regard to the Emotional Stability category, descriptions of children's resilience or good control of emotions refer to the high end of emotional reactivity, while frequent crying, sensitivity and reactivity to stress represent its low end. Likewise, the descriptions of self-assurance or self-certainty, and lacking self-confidence or feelings of insecurity characterize high and low end of the self-confidence, respectively. Finally, anxiety/fear at its high end denotes descriptions of children not exhibiting lots of fears, who are relaxed and calm, whereas the subcategory accounts for portrays of worrisome, tense, and nervous children at the opposite end.

Across the age samples from seven countries, the vast majority of child characteristics were coded into the categories of the FFM (Kohnstamm et al., 1998). In general, Emotional Stability was (along with Conscientiousness) the least salient of the five main categories for parents describing their children (from about 7% to 10% of descriptions) but it was nevertheless more capacious than any of the additional categories outside the FFM. The differences among the countries were small with respect to overall (high and low end) percentages of descriptions coded for Emotional Stability and its subcategories; the Emotional Reactivity subcategory received most descriptors across the countries, and over 70% of child characteristics in the Emotional Stability category were coded low, i.e. in terms of instability, reactivity and negative affectivity (Angleitner et al., 1998). Using a more elaborate methodology based on a multiple-informant approach (mothers, fathers, day-care teachers), and extended to descriptions of infants and toddlers, very similar results were demonstrated in Slovenia (Zupančič, 2001, 2004; Zupančič & Kavčič, 2002). Figure 1 displays average proportions of overall Slovene descriptions at the category and subcategory level of the Emotional Stability category for independent maternal and paternal reports on their infants/toddlers (1 to 3 year-olds) and preschoolers aged from 3 to 7 years (Zupančič, 2004).

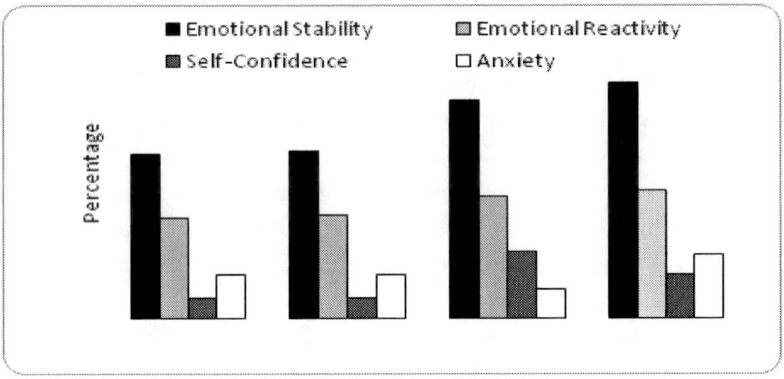

Figure 1. Average proportions of overall maternal and paternal descriptions of infants/toddlers (I/T) and preschoolers (PS) in the Emotional Stability category and its subcategories (data from Zupančič, 2004).

The fact that the caregivers across countries (Angleitner et al., 1998; Zupančič, 2001, 2004; Zupančič & Kavčič, 2002) describe children of different ages (Slotboom, Havill, Pavlopoulos, & De Fruyt, 1998; Zupančič, 2004; Zupančič & Kavčič, 2002) mostly in terms of emotional instability or neuroticism rather than stable and confident characteristics is consistent with the temperament literature in which negatively valued constructs are used, and with the frequency of terms for emotional stability in the adult lexicon. As noted in many languages, much fewer words in the lexicons connote emotional stability than neuroticism (see Angleitner et al., 1998). It can further be assumed from the free descriptive studies of children that the majority of caregivers are not concerned about negative reactivity, anxiety, fear or lack of self-confidence in children since these terms are seldom used in descriptions. The good-functioning emotional characteristics of normative children may be taken for granted and thus, less likely mentioned during the interviews (Angleitner et al., 1998; Havill et al., 1994). In addition, typical children may be expected to be more reactive emotionally and more poorly regulated than mature individuals. The adults may consider relatively instable behavioral patterns common for all children and therefore, not relevant for social comparisons. Consequently, characteristics of emotional instability may be less likely stated as salient child features than those classified within the other four FFM categories (Havill et al., 1994; Zupančič, 2004).

In general, child descriptions concerning the overall Emotional Stability category were as salient for the Slovene infants/toddlers as for the preschoolers (Zupančič, 2004) and no age differences (3 to 12 years) at the high end of the category were found within the multi-national project (Slotboom et al., 1998). However, the parents in Belgium, the Netherlands, and Slovenia used somewhat more descriptions referring to overall emotional instability, especially emotional reactivity, when describing older children as compared to younger ones (Slotboom et al., 1998; Zupančič, 2004). The traits parents come to see in their children may, along with the saliency of the traits, depend on parental expectations about what traits are important for children at different ages in their particular culture. Perhaps parents in the three aforementioned countries expect a more rapid emotional maturation in their children than parents in other countries of the multi-national project; the former may therefore, talk more about the traits referring to emotional reactivity with increasing age of children because more emotionally stable responses that were expected to occur are still absent in their children.

Neuroticism as Defined by the New Generation Measures of Child FFM Personality Traits

Specific inventories to assess child personality traits were constructed relying on the findings of the free-descriptive research. They cover a wide range of individual differences that are observed salient by the caregivers and include items generated from parental natural language. Two such instruments were developed, the Hierarchical Personality Inventory for Children (HiPIC; Mervielde & De Fruyt, 2002) and the Inventory of Child Individual Differences (ICID; Halverson et al., 2003). They share substantial commonalities concerning the item content and capture a variety of similar specific trait scales (labeled somewhat differently), which are organized around the FFM broad personality traits. Yet, the inventories differ in several respects. Most notably, the HiPIC is targeted at the primary school children aged from 6 to 12 years (Mervielde & De Fruyt, 2002), whereas the ICID is constructed as an age- and culture neutral instrument (for details see Halverson et al., 2003), applicable from at least age 3 through adolescence (Halverson et al., 2003; Knyazev et al., 2008; Slobodskaya, 2007; Zupančič & Kavčič, 2004, 2009).

There is also a discrepancy in the structure of neuroticism as measured by the HiPIC and the ICID, which may depend on idiosyncratic properties of the instruments. The dimension in HiPIC (labeled Emotional Stability) is defined by low anxiety (e.g., the child is not quick to worry about things) and self-confidence (e.g., takes decisions easily), whereas (low) shyness (e.g., tries to establish contact with new class-fellows) and (low) irritability (e.g., not quick to take offence) are the constituents of extraversion and agreeableness (labeled Benevolence), respectively (Mervielde & De Fruyt, 2002). However, the ICID specific traits (also referred to as mid-level traits) of fearful/insecure (corresponding to anxiety and low self-confidence in the HiPIC), and shy are consistently represented in the dimension of neuroticism (Halverson et al., 2003; Knyazev et al., 2008; Zupančič & Kavčič, 2004, 2009; Zupančič et al., 2009); also, the ICID specific trait of negative affect (resembling irritability in the HiPIC) usually co-varies with both neuroticism and disagreeableness (or low agreeableness). We introduce the three specific traits, fearful/insecure, shy, and negative affect and the broad dimension of neuroticism as measured by the ICID more closely because the findings in the following sections are largely drawn from studies using this inventory.

Among the consistent ICID constituents of neuroticism, fearfulness/insecurity characterizes children who are easily upset, tend to be apprehensive, distressed, quick to panic, feel insecure, lack confidence, and are afraid of lots of things, whereas shyness describes children who are socially reticent, slow to warm up to new people or social situations, tend to be withdrawn, quiet, and often prefer to be alone. The specific trait of negative affect features children experiencing lots of negative emotions in interpersonal situations, who are irritable, moody, get angry easily, quick tempered. Negative affectivity shows stronger links with disagreeableness than neuroticism when all of the 15 specific ICID traits are factor analyzed; in this case, an invariant four-factor solution (openness does not emerge) across children's ages and informants providing the personality ratings is obtained (Zupančič & Kavčič, 2009). However, when the mid-level traits of considerate and compliant are omitted due to their low discriminability, negative affect is more closely linked with neuroticism than disagreeableness; in this case, the five-factors are clearly recovered across child ages, gender, informants, and countries (Knyazev et al., 2008), a result similar to the original US validation study with the compliant mid-level scale dropped (Halverson et al., 2003). Because negative affectivity as captured by the ICID can be empirically subsumed by the broad neuroticism or disagreeableness, we address three specific traits (fearful/insecure, shy, and negative affect) along with the broad ICID neuroticism trait in most parts of the remaining paper, which is focused on the period of early childhood.

Can we reliably measure neuroticism and its specific trait constituents over early childhood? Although research in this developmental period has been scarce to date, compelling evidence has been provided on the reliability of Neuroticism scales as assessed by different informants, using diverse measures and referring to target children in several countries (e.g., Abe & Izard, 1999; Asendorpf & Van Aken, 2003; De Pauw et al., 2009; Grist & McCord, 2010; Halverson et al., 2003; Knyazev et al., 2008; Lamb et al., 2002; Zupančič & Kavčič, 2004, Zupančič et al., 2009). Specifically, the internal coherence (α) for the broad ICID Neuroticism scale in our standardization sample ranged from .84 to .88 across gender and age (3, 4, 5, 6 years) of the target children, and the informants providing the child ratings (mothers, fathers, preschool and school teachers). The internal reliability of the two consistent constituent traits of neuroticism, and of negative affect obtained with the same samples was also satisfactory, ranging from .64 to .78 for fearful/insecure, from .70 to .87 for shy, and from .80 to .91 for negative affect (Zupančič & Kavčič, 2009).

Types of Developmental Consistency in Neuroticism over Early Childhood

Developmentally, it is crucial to explore different types of temporal consistency of personality traits in order to explain how individuals change or remain the same in response to changing developmental ecologies. In order to provide this information, we investigated several aspects of child personality consistency in a longitudinal study using the ICID (Zupančič & Kavčič, 2007, 2009; Zupančič et al., 2009). Data on child neuroticism, its constituent traits, and negative affect were collected from mothers, fathers and (pre)school teachers of children at ages of 3, 4, 5 and 6 years. To our knowledge, this is the only follow-up study of personality traits focused specifically on the development over early childhood. Thus, we draw on our own empirical work based on questionnaire data by multiple informants and present an overview of several types of developmental (mean-level, individual-level and rank-order) and cross-informant consistency in neuroticism, its specific trait constituents, and negative affect over early childhood.

Mean-Level Consistency in Ratings of Early Childhood Neuroticism

Mean-level or normative consistency refers to continuity in the average trait level of a population over time. The average level of a trait is typically assessed by mean-level differences in a given trait over time, which indicates whether an age-sample as a whole is increasing or decreasing on the trait (Roberts & DelVecchio, 2000).

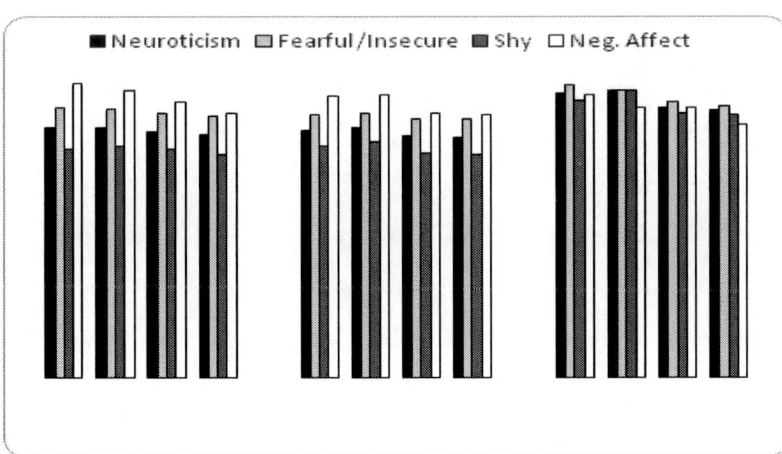

Figure 2. Mean scores (on a scale from 1 to 7, with 1=characteristic present in a child much less than in the average same-age peer, 4=same, 7= much more) for neuroticism, its constituents, and negative affect as obtained by mother, father and (pre)school teacher ratings of children over early childhood.

Accounting for one-year time intervals between consecutive measurements, no significant mean-level change in maternal and paternal ratings of neuroticism and its specific trait constituents (fearful/insecure, and shy) was revealed from child age 3 through 6 (see Figure 2 for mean ICID scores). A continual and small decrease in mean levels of neuroticism and its marker traits was noted according to teacher ratings of the same children (Zupančič & Kavčič, 2009). Concerning negative affect, a small age decrease was observed across the observer ratings. All of the significant age changes were small, with age explaining up to 4% of variance in adult reports of children's neuroticism or negative affect. The small size of age changes is, in general, consistent with findings of other cross-sectional ICID studies on age differences in personality between early and middle childhood (Halverson, 2003; Slobodskaya, 2005; Zupančič, Gril, & Kavčič, 2006). The estimated change as measured with the ICID may be somewhat deflated since the informants may have compared the target children to their peers of the same age.

The mean-level changes can be considered to result from maturational processes and environmental influences shared by the sample of children (Robins, Fraley, Roberts, & Trzesniewski, 2001). Though small, the observed developmental change in neuroticism and negative affect may point to increasing maturity as young children become more proficient in emotional regulation and general psychological functioning. Maturation promotes the development of many competencies (e.g., social skills, coping strategies, capacities to regulate emotion and delay gratification), whereas (pre)school and home environment provides age-specific pressure for change (Zupančič et al., 2009).

Rank-Order Consistency in Ratings of Early Childhood Neuroticism

Rank-order consistency reflects the degree to which the relative ordering of individuals on a given trait is maintained over time. This type of consistency is theoretically and statistically distinct from mean-level consistency. Rank-ordering of individuals on a trait could change substantially over time but without any aggregate increases/decreases (the number of individuals who decreased offset the number of those who increased). Similarly, a population could increase substantially on a trait, but the rank-ordering of individuals would be maintained if everyone increased by the same amount (Roberts & DelVecchio, 2000).

Meta-analyses of studies using various temperament/personality measures and methods of assessments (questionnaires, observations, interviews) in early childhood, including infancy and toddlerhood, showed modest rank-order consistency of temperament traits during the first three years of life after birth and then an increase towards moderate levels of stability during the preschool years. The mean rank-order consistency of negative affectivity, for example, ranged from .35 to .41 (Roberts & DelVecchio, 2000). Regarding early childhood neuroticism, the findings of our longitudinal studies (Zupančič & Kavčič, 2007, 2009; Zupančič et al., 2009) showed statistically significant temporal stability in rank-order of neuroticism and its specific traits (see Table 1).

Table 1. Rank-Order Stability (r) of Neuroticism, its Constituents, and Negative Affect as Rated by Mothers, Fathers and Teachers over Early Childhood

Rater	*N*	Fearful/ Insecure	Negative Affect	Shy	Neuroticism
From child age 3 to 4 years					
Mothers	294	0.60***	0.62***	0.56***	0.63***
Fathers	256	0.51***	0.51***	0.48***	0.52***
Teachers	287	0.49***	0.48***	0.54***	0.55***
From child age 4 to 5 years					
Mothers	273	0.65***	0.64***	0.63***	0.69***
Fathers	262	0.61***	0.62***	0.63***	0.65***
Teachers	286	0.51***	0.48***	0.52***	0.49***
From child age 5 to 6 years					
Mothers	216	0.67***	0.74***	0.68***	0.71***
Fathers	201	0.64***	0.67***	0.68***	0.70***
Teachers	217	0.22**	0.34***	0.19**	0.21**
From child age 3 to 5 years					
Mothers	276	0.59***	0.56***	0.56***	0.62***
Fathers	258	0.60***	0.49***	0.51***	0.59***
Teachers	321	0.27***	0.37***	0.36***	0.34***
From child age 4 to 6 years					
Mothers	202	0.58***	0.60***	0.59***	0.61***
Fathers	188	0.62***	0.63***	0.56***	0.61***
Teachers	194	0.26***	0.42***	0.29***	0.28***
From child age 3 to 6 years					
Mothers	202	0.51***	0.48***	0.56***	0.57***
Fathers	187	0.46***	0.48***	0.54***	0.55***
Teachers	212	0.21**	0.26***	0.27***	0.26***

Note. ** $p < 0.01$, *** $p < 0.001$

The stability coefficients varied in size, depending on the informants providing the child personality ratings: The estimated stability of maternal and paternal reports was moderate to high over time (between one-, two- and three-year time intervals), while the stability of teacher reports was low to moderate. Using the HiPIC, Prinzie and Deković (2008) also reported on lower estimates (moderate) of rank-order stability of teacher reported neuroticism in school-aged children as compared to the stability of parental reports across the same age range (De Fruyt, Bartels, Van Leeuwen, De Clercq, Decuyper, & Mervielde, 2006).

As displayed in Table 1, our study showed a slight increase in temporal stability of parental ratings of child neuroticism and the three specific traits with age of the target children. However, the lower rank-order stability of scores derived by teachers between child ages 5 and 6 years as compared to previous waves of the study may be due to the children's entry into compulsory school at age 6; the children thus, changed the educational setting (preschool vs. school) and each child was rated by a different teacher at age 6 than age 5 (lots of the target children remained in the same group with the same teacher over the preschool years). Furthermore, the temporal stability coefficients were inversely related to the time interval between consecutive measurements – the rank-order stability of trait ratings was higher for shorter than longer time intervals, which is consistent with previous studies of personality stability over time (e.g., Roberts & DelVecchio, 2000). Also, the temporal stability was stronger for the same rater-scores than for the cross-ratings (Zupančič et al., 2009), suggesting that the same-rater bias may slightly inflate the rank-order stability estimates. Conversely, the rank-order stability coefficients may be underestimated for neuroticism and its specific traits when reports by others instead of self-ratings are used because these traits probably become more covert over age and may be thus, subjected to less accurate assessments than other personality traits (e.g., extraversion, agreeableness).

Several mechanisms may contribute to the rank-order stability of child personality over time (for review, see Roberts, Wood, & Caspi, 2008), for example, the consistency in children's environment (our target participants remained in the same homes with both caregivers and attended the same preschools before the school entry in the course of our investigation), genetic factors, and person–environment transactions (e.g., a shy child may avoid peer interactions and consequently get fewer opportunities to develop good socials skills). On the other hand, temporal stability of neuroticism and its constituents is not perfect. Changes in rank-ordering result from maturational or experiential factors that affect individuals differentially and from measurement error (Roberts & DelVecchio, 2000). Temporal stability in neuroticism and its specific traits thus, allows for a noteworthy change during early childhood.

Individual-Level Consistency in Ratings of Early Childhood Neuroticism

Individual level consistency/change refers to the magnitude of increase or decrease observed on a given trait in each individual over time. Individuals can significantly change (increase or decrease) in a trait even though mean-level comparisons show no normative changes in the whole sample. We used the RCI (the Reliable Change Index) scores in order to determine, how many children changed or did not change significantly in neuroticism, its specific constituent traits, and negative affect as rated by their parents (maternal and paternal ratings aggregated) and teachers (Zupančič & Kavčič, 2007). The RCI scores (Jacobson & Truax, 1991) provide a measure of the change in standardized units, the direction of the change, and whether it is reliable (Zahra & Hedge, 2010).

The results presented in Table 2 show that a vast majority of children (over 90%) did not change significantly in neuroticism and its specific traits. Prinzie and Deković (2008) report on similar results, with 6% of school-aged children changing significantly in teacher-rated emotional stability over a three-year-time period. Consistent with the normative (small) decrease in neuroticism (teacher ratings only) and negative affect established in our study, children displayed a reliable age-related decrease rather than increase in neuroticism, fearfulness/insecurity, negative affect, and shyness. Nevertheless, a few children changed significantly in these traits in the opposite direction, i.e. their scores obtained by the ratings of adults increased reliably over time.

If individual-level change were random, we would expect roughly 2.5% of the sample to increase, 2.5% to decrease, and 95% not to change reliably (Roberts, Caspi, & Moffitt, 2001). We can therefore, conclude that somewhat greater than chance levels of change occurring at the individual level emerged for all of the respective traits and across the informant ratings in our study, even though the parental reports showed a significant mean-level change in negative affect only. Accordingly, the teacher reports revealed somewhat more individual level change in the respective children's traits than parental reports. This pattern could, in part, reflect the fact that the children were not assessed by the same teachers across the waves of the study. Higher individual stability of parent-rated child neuroticism and the respective marker traits could also be due to a tendency for parents to model a stereotyped view of their child that is resistant to change over time (Prinzie & Deković, 2008).

Table 2. Percentage of Children Changing Significantly in Scores of Neuroticism (N), its Constituents, and Negative Affect (Parent and Teacher Ratings) over Early Childhood

	Teachers				Parents			
	Fearful/ Insecure	Negative Affect	Shy	N	Fearful/ Insecure	Negative Affect	Shy	N
From 3 to 4 years								
Increase	4	4	4	5	2	2	2	3
Decrease	3	2	2	3	2	4	2	2
Change	8	6	6	8	4	6	5	5
From 4 to 5 years								
Increase	1	3	1	1	3	2	4	2
Decrease	5	5	4	5	4	4	5	4
Change	6	8	6	6	7	5	8	7
From 5 to 6 years								
Increase	6	3	4	4	2	2	2	2
Decrease	3	4	1	2	5	5	4	4
Change	9	7	6	6	7	7	6	6
From 3 to 5 years								
Increase	2	3	2	2	3	2	4	3
Decrease	6	5	4	4	3	5	4	4
Change	8	8	5	6	6	7	8	7
From 4 to 6 years								
Increase	5	3	2	3	4	2	2	4
Decrease	5	5	4	5	5	6	6	5
Change	10	7	6	8	9	8	9	9
From 3 to 6 years								
Increase	3	1	3	3	2	3	4	2
Decrease	5	5	5	5	4	6	4	4
Change	8	7	8	8	6	8	8	6

Cross-Informant Consistency in Neuroticism in Early Childhood

In addition to temporal stability, consistency in personality traits can be assessed across different raters or contexts concurrently. The multi-informant design of our study (Zupančič & Kavčič, 2009) enabled us to investigate: (a) the mean-level consistency of ratings of child neuroticism, fearfulness/insecurity, shyness, and negative affect across the informants (mother, fathers, teachers), which reflects systematic similarities or differences in perceptions/assessments of a given child trait by different groups of informants, and (b) the rank-order consistency in the respective trait ratings, referring to the degree of agreement between pairs of informants on trait expression in the same child.

Parent and (pre)school teacher reports on children's neuroticism and its marker traits differed significantly across the waves of our study. The parents (both mothers and fathers) reported on more socially desirable (lower) levels of neuroticism (small to moderate effect size), fearfulness/insecurity (small effect size), and shyness (moderate to large effect size) in their children than teachers (see also Figure 2). However, the differences between informant ratings declined with the children's age. With regard to negative affectivity, significant differences between the informant groups were obtained at child age 6 only. The parents rated their children somewhat higher in negative affect than the teachers. Across the children's ages, the spouses did not differ significantly in their mean levels of child personality ratings under our inquiry. The differences in child trait ratings between parents and teachers could be due to (Zupančič & Kavčič, 2007; Zupančič et al., 2009):

- Differences in contexts (home vs. (pre)school) in which the informants observe children; the children behave differently across different contexts (e.g., Harris, 1998);
- Differences in criteria used to judge children's personality characteristics; teachers are more likely to compare the target child's characteristics to a larger group of his/her same-aged peers than parents because the former interact with groups of children on daily basis;
- Differences in relationships between informants and children, and differences in social roles the informants occupy in relation to children (parent vs. teacher). Characteristics of parent-child relationships vs. educator-child relationships could, for example, contribute to more positively biased parental than teacher reports on

child neuroticism and its marker traits (though this is not evidenced in ratings of negative affect) due to the own-child enhancement effect.

The factors suggested may also help explain the similarities in mean ratings of child neuroticism (and its specific traits) between parents. Both mothers and fathers report on their child from similar (parental) role perspectives and relationships with the child, observe the child in the same (home) context, and have similar criteria available to compare the child characteristics to those of his/her age-peers. Nevertheless, the differences revealed between parental and teacher mean-level scores do not imply more accurate ratings of child personality by either group of informants.

A substantial interrater agreement on relative child trait standings was found in our studies (Zupančič & Kavčič, 2009; Zupančič et al., 2009) with respect to neuroticism, its constituent straits, and negative affect (see Table 3). Concurrent cross-informant rank-order stability in the observed child neuroticism traits, and negative affect is consistently stronger between the spouses than between parents and teachers. The agreement between mothers and fathers is high and agreement between parents and teachers of same children ranges from low to moderate in size across early childhood, whereas the agreement between different teachers in school is moderate. Parent and teacher assessments of children depend on different information gathered in different settings and different roles the observers occupy, which results in them taking different perspectives on children's characteristics. Moreover, the spouses communicate on their child more than they do with the teacher. Nevertheless, when different adults observe children in a similar context and from a similar perspective they agree in their ratings of child neuroticism and its specific traits to a greater extent as compared to the cross-context/perspective agreements. Along with previously documented high agreement between mothers and fathers (De Fruyt & Vollrath, 2003) and modest associations between maternal and teacher ratings (Barbaranelli et al., 2003) of school-aged children's neuroticism, our findings suggest that the ratings of child traits depend on the context in which child behavior is observed and the informants' perspective. However, personality does not exist only in the eyes of the informant as suggested by significant agreements between raters, even across different contexts.

Table 3. Inter-Rater Agreement in Ratings of Child Neuroticism, its Constituents, and Negative Affect over Early Childhood

Pairs of Raters	N	Fearful/ Insecure	Negative Affect	Shy	Neuroticism
Child age 3 years					
Mother – Father	281	0.63***	0.56***	0.65***	0.68***
Mother – PS Teacher	307	0.28***	0.15*	0.25***	0.28***
Father – PS Teacher	288	0.18**	0.12*	0.22***	0.23***
Child age 4 years					
Mother – Father	276	0.62***	0.55***	0.60***	0.63***
Mother – PS Teacher	270	0.31***	0.18**	0.38***	0.38***
Father – PS Teacher	259	0.24***	0.17**	0.28***	0.28***
Child age 5 years					
Mother – Father	281	0.68***	0.62***	0.69***	0.71***
Mother – PS Teacher	303	0.31***	0.24***	0.30***	0.34***
Father – PS Teacher	286	0.28***	0.15*	0.25***	0.29***
Child age 6 years					
Mother – Father	259	0.66***	0.68***	0.70***	0.72***
Mother – Teacher	251	0.25***	0.17**	0.23***	0.25***
Father – Teacher	231	0.20**	0.24***	0.21**	0.21**
A Teacher – Teacher	275	0.49***	0.59***	0.53***	0.53***

Note. PS stands for Preschool; A Teacher refers to the assistant school teacher and Teacher to the primary school teacher. Both teachers are present in the classroom of Slovene first grade of basic compulsory school.

* $p < 0.05$, ** $p < 0.01$, *** $p < 0.001$.

Gender Differences in Early Childhood Neuroticism

In general, gender differences in neuroticism among adults were well documented, with females scoring higher than males across age-groups, countries, and methods of assessment (e.g., Feingold, 1994; Lynn & Martin, 1997; McCrae, Terracciano et al., 2005). A meta-analysis of ratings of 3 month to 13-year-olds further suggested small gender effects for temperamental difficulty favoring boys, and fear as well as shyness favoring girls (Else-Quest, Hyde, Goldsmith, & Van Hulle, 2006). The expected gender differences in neuroticism as measured by the ICID were also demonstrated for parental reports of 3 to 14 year old Chinese children/adolescents but no significant gender differences emerged among the US and Greek children

(Halverson, 2003). Similarly, results of several studies employing observational data or parent ratings indicated no significant gender differences in overall shyness (e.g., Bishop et al., 2003; Findlay et al., 2009). Small and mostly non-significant gender differences in the ICID neuroticism and its specific traits (including negative affect) were revealed in a comparative study of Slovene and Russian cross-sectional data; significant gender differences were inconsistently distributed across the age-groups from toddlerhood through adolescence and were mainly present in Slovenia. When parental ratings of boys and girls differed significantly, the differences even appeared in the opposite direction than expected, except for negative affect; the boys were rated higher in negative affectivity but also in fear, shyness, and overall neuroticism than were the girls (Zupančič, Slobodskaya, & Knyazev, 2008).

In addition to the cross-sectional comparative study of pre-adult gender differences in personality (Zupančič et al., 2008), we explored personality gender differences in a longitudinal study of children with data provided by multiple-informants (Zupančič & Kavčič, 2005, 2009). Ratings of mothers, fathers, and teachers yielded significant, though small gender differences in child neuroticism (see Figure 3), its marker traits, and negative affect rather consistently across early childhood. Consonant with cross-sectional research indicating higher levels of neuroticism in parental ratings of Slovene boys as compared to girls (Puklek & Gril, 1999; Zupančič et al., 2006; Zupančič et al., 2008), the boys ($N = 128$ to 166) of our longitudinal inquiry were perceived by the adults somewhat higher in neuroticism traits (overall neuroticism, fearful/insecure, and shy) than the girls ($N = 137$ to 166) but mothers and teachers assigned somewhat more negative affectivity to 5- and 6-year-old boys than girls. It appears plausible that the Slovene adults emphasize emotional stability in girls more often than in boys because boys are expected to be stable according to their gender role, while the emotional stability in girls is attributed to their personality.

The gender differences evidenced in our early childhood research (Zupančič & Kavčič, 2005, 2009) were already present in 3-year-olds but did not increase with the child age as would be expected from the biosocial hypothesis (for an overview, see Feingold, 1994): If the social-cultural factors augmented inherent gender differences over time, the gender differences in neuroticism, its marker traits, and negative affect would tend to increase. Besides, it is noteworthy that the gender differences in adult-rated child neuroticism, its marker traits, and negative affect were small in size, a finding documented across the studies (Else-Quest, 2006; Halverson, 2003; Zupančič et al., 2008). Nevertheless, the effect of gender may be underestimated in research relying on adult reports because the informants may assess the target child's characteristics with regard to his/her peers of the same gender. Along with biological and socio-cultural influences that presumably shape personality by gender, the informant response bias may also contribute to gender differences in child personality. When the parent- and adolescent ICID self-reports were compared, for example, no significant gender differences were shown in neuroticism, shyness, and negative affect but the differences in fearfulness/insecurity appeared in the expected direction, i.e. favoring girls (Zupančič et al., 2008).

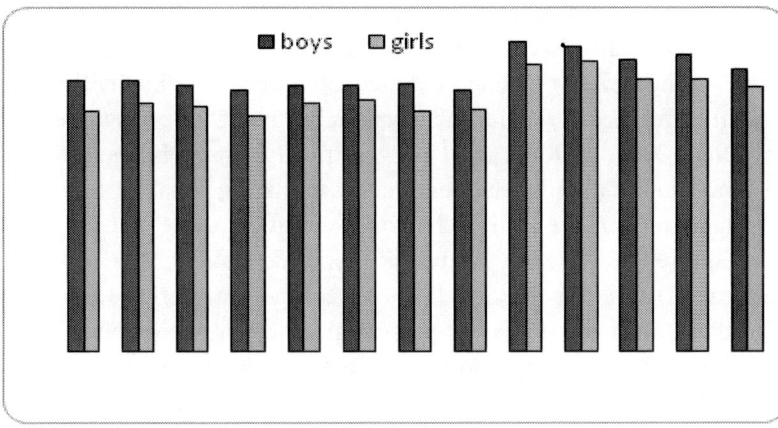

Figure 3. Mean scores (on a scale from 1 to 7; 1=characteristic present in a child much less than in the average same-age peer, 4=same, 7= much more) by maternal, paternal and teacher ratings of neuroticism in boys and girls over early childhood.

EARLY CHILDHOOD NEUROTICISM AND ITS BEHAVIORAL EXPRESSIONS

How is child neuroticism manifested in developmental ecologies over early childhood? Most notably, adult perceptions of child neuroticism show consistent concurrent and longitudinal associations with expressions of internalizing behavior and difficulties in social relationships across multiple settings but may also protect children against development of externalizing problems (e.g., De Pauw et al., 2009; Slobodskaya, 2007; Zupančič & Kavčič, 2004, 2007, 2009, 2011). Adding to the studies in the field, our research suggests that neuroticism also shapes early sibling relationships (Kavčič &

Zupančič, 2006, 2011), socially competent behavior in educational settings (Zupančič & Kavčič, 2007, 2009), and predicts developmental trajectories of internalizing behavior, and externalizing behavior across early childhood (Kavčič, Podlesek, & Zupančič, 2012).

Neuroticism and Social Adjustment

The following findings are based on our questionnaire studies, employing the ICID and controlling for the same-rater bias. Neuroticism (defined by fearful/insecure, and shy trait constituents) at ages 3, 4, 5, and 6 years (*N*s from 256 to 331) as observed in home (parent reports) or educational settings (teacher ratings) both contemporaneously and longitudinally predicted individual differences in children's social adjustment in (pre)school (Zupančič & Kavčič, 2007, 2009, 2011). Specifically, associations with social competence, internalizing behavior, and externalizing behavior as measured by the Social Competence and Behavior Evaluation scale (SCBE - Slovene version; LaFreniere, Dumas, Zupančič, Gril, & Kavčič, 2001) were clearly demonstrated. In short, the SCBE social competence reflects joyful, secure, tolerant child behavior in his/her preschool group or school class, integration into the peer group, calm and prosocial behavior toward peers, cooperative and age-appropriate autonomy in relation to teachers; the SCBE internalizing behavior captures expressions of depression and anxiety, relative isolation in a peer group, and dependence on teachers, whereas externalizing behavior describes expressions of anger, aggression and egotistical behavior toward peers, and oppositional behavior in relation to teachers. A large amount of our findings can be generalized as follows:

1. Concurrent predictions of social adjustment measures over the preschool years (ages 3, 4, and 5) through the beginning of the first grade of elementary school (age 6) are stronger than the longitudinal ones though both types of predictions are consistently significant. The finding may be attributed to less than perfect temporal stability of the observed child neuroticism and social behavior (e.g., Zupančič & Kavčič, 2007; Zupančič et al., 2009). In addition, neuroticism and internalizing behavior were unambiguously documented to show concomitant change over early childhood (Kavčič et al., 2012).
2. Teacher or assistant teacher reports on child neuroticism are more predictive of his/her social adjustment as observed by assistant

teachers or teachers than parental assessments of child neuroticism. This is probably due to the fact that the teacher and assistant teacher ratings of both neuroticism and adjustment (although cross-rated) were based on observations of children in the same context (educational) and from similar role perspectives. The teachers also interact with a much broader range of children than parents and presumably have more expertise regarding normative development and individual differences among children, which may contribute to a greater accuracy of teacher- as compared to parent ratings of child personality.

3. Child neuroticism (parent or teacher-rated) shows a strong incremental validity over and beyond a set of family variables (parental education, parent-reported authoritative parenting, power assertion, ineffective control, and stimulation of child cognitive development) and preschool attendance (age of entry, alternative types of care). Although educational background of the family and parenting over early childhood are linked to child outcomes, the associations with child social development are generally modest (except in severely adverse families) (e.g., Bradley, Corwyn, Burchinall, Pipes McAdoo, & Garcia Coll, 2001; Miller, Tserakhawa, & Miller, 2011), especially with children's out-of-home social behavior (Harris, 1998).
4. Adult reports on child neuroticism predict measures of social adjustment in (pre)school differentially. Parent- and teacher-rated child neuroticism is consistently and most strongly (both concurrently and longitudinally) related to internalizing behavior in educational settings. The trait and its constituents are assumed to predispose children to inhibit their approach towards others (Caspi & Silva, 1995; De Pauw & Mervielde, 2010) and engagement in peer groups, which may contribute to the emotionally instable children being overlooked and ignored by their peers as reflected in high SCBE internalizing scores used in our studies. Individual differences in neuroticism (or any other trait) further play an important role in a cumulative process of person–environment transactions (e.g., Caspi, 2000). Individuals differing in neuroticism may interpret and react differently to similar experiences, evoke distinctive responses from others, and actively tend to select or create different environments for themselves. Children prone to fearfulness, social inhibition, and lacking of self-confidence may thus, tend to interpret peer behavior as overly

> competent, dominant or even threatening and/or frequently feel too embarrassed to actively engage in social interactions; they may evoke peer neglect and overprotectiveness by adults (Gallagher, 2002; Rubin, Nelson, Hastings, & Asendorpf, 1999) due to their passive, meek, non-assertive and non-aggressive interactive style (Caspi & Silva. 1995); finally, they may tend to recreate for themselves the same social conditions (staying aside the peers and rely on adults) over and over again.

More emotionally instable 6-year-olds (according to parent reports) in our studies tend to be viewed as less socially competent in school, too. Children who are easily upset, slow to warm up to new people or social situations, tend to be apprehensive, distressed, withdrawn, quiet and lack self-confidence may have difficulties in initiating and maintaining satisfying interactions and relationships with others, which puts them at disadvantage in gaining social knowledge, social skills (Gomes & Livesey, 2008) and social coping strategies (Findlay et al., 2009), the important components of socially competent behavior.

Besides the undesirable behavioral manifestations of neuroticism, we also evidenced consistent but weaker and negative associations between neuroticism and externalizing behavior. The children who were perceived more emotionally stable by their parents and teachers were more likely to exhibit externalizing behaviors in (pre)school. Similarly to the findings drawn from temperament research (e.g., Kochanska, 1997; Rothbart & Putnam, 2002), fearfulness, anxiety, insecurity and shyness as captured by the ICID neuroticism seem to predispose children toward inhibition of impulsive responses (e.g., aggressive) and guilt-proneness which promotes the development of rule-abiding behavior.

Neuroticism and Trajectories of Social Adjustment

Nevertheless, not only baselines (as obtained by single-measurements) but also the change in neuroticism (teacher ratings) over early childhood was shown to be related to the development of internalizing behavior and externalizing behavior in a random sample of 304 children attending public preschools prior to school entry (Kavčič et al., 2012). The change in the development of neuroticism was clearly reflected in the trajectory of internalizing behavior and also predicted the trajectory of externalizing behavior. An increase in the rank in internalizing behavior over child ages 3 to 6 was related to an increase in the rank in neuroticism, and an increase in the rank in externalizing behavior was predicted by a decrease in the rank of neuroticism. The trait may be viewed as predisposing children towards overt expressions of anxiety, sadness, behavioral inhibition in social interactions and novel situations, and over-reliance on adults that characterize the cluster of internalizing behavior. The reviews by De Pauw and Mervielde (2010), and Shiner (2006) concluded that early child fearfulness, insecurity and shyness are manifested in withdrawal-related behavioral responses. Such responses were reflected through poor peer engagement of the children rated high in neuroticism in our research, their cautious behavior in the preschool group or school class, wariness in challenging situations, and dependence on adults (teachers).

On the other hand, the significant role of decreasing neuroticism in the development of externalizing behavior (Kavčič et al., 2012) suggested that low levels of fear, worry, anxiety, and social wariness may predispose youngsters towards aggression, especially in an instrumental (proactive) manner (De Pauw & Mervielde, 2010).

The concomitant changes in developmental trajectories of neuroticism, internalizing behavior and externalizing behavior, however, do not preclude bi-directional influences between the trait and social adjustments. The early emerging individual differences in neuroticism may shape the behavioral outcomes but social (mal)adaptations may also shape typical ways of feeling, thinking and behaving. In order to explore the direction of short-term longitudinal relations between child neuroticism (teacher ratings) and internalizing behavior (assistant teacher reports), we tested the paths from neuroticism at age 5 to internalizing behavior at age 6 (N = 240), and from internalizing behavior at age 5 to neuroticism at age 6, while controlling for concurrent associations between the respective variables at both ages, and temporal stability of both measures. Children's dispositional tendencies towards neuroticism were demonstrated more likely to influence subsequent internalizing behavior than vice versa. Child neuroticism as viewed by preschool teachers at age 5 directly influenced the assistant school teacher assessments of child internalizing behavior one year later but the cross-lagged path from earlier internalizing behavior to later neuroticism was non-significant (Zupančič, Podlesek, & Kavčič, 2012). The finding is consistent with the Five-Factor theory which posits that personality traits represent endogenous dispositions that follow intrinsic paths of development (McCrae et al., 2000). According to this theory, the traits are proposed to affect behavioral outcomes, whereas the behavioral (mal)adjustments are not expected to shape personality. Of course the result of our study (Zupančič et al., 2012) is limited to the constructs as measured by the ICID neuroticism and the SCBE internalizing behavior over a relatively short time period, and the cross-lagged design does not necessarily imply a cause-effect relationship.

Neuroticism and Sibling Relationships

In addition to the meaningful links of neuroticism with social adjustment, our research documents that parent-rated child neuroticism is predictive of sibling relationships over early childhood both concurrently and over a one-year-time period (Kavčič & Zupančič, 2006, 2011). With sibling dyads (*N*s from 66 to 100; an average age gap of 26 months, with *SD* of 9 months), sets of parental cross-ratings (maternal or paternal) of both children's neuroticism were significantly (at best moderately) linked to father- or mother-perceived sibling conflict. The higher the younger and/or the older sibling's level of neuroticism perceived by one parent the more conflict in sibling interactions was observed by the other parent. Social inhibition, fear, anxiety, insecurity of emotionally instable children may be obvious in their non-assertive, timid, hesitant, and withdrawn behaviors during interactions with peers and authority figures (teachers) in structured social settings such as preschool groups or school classes. But those children may feel more relaxed, confident, self-assertive, dominant and less withdrawn during interactions with their well-known siblings in secure home settings, and may thus express their dissatisfaction, frustration, and moodiness in a proactive manner, which may lead to sibling conflict.

A higher level of neuroticism in older siblings was further associated with lower levels of parent-observed warmth between siblings and the older child's personality also appeared to have a somewhat stronger role in both parent-observed sibling conflict and warmth than the younger child's personality. Although the older child's parent-rated neuroticism as compared to the ratings of the younger child was suggested to contribute more to the perceived quality of sibling relationships, which is perhaps due to a more active and initiatory role of the older than younger child during sibling social exchanges (e.g., Dunn, 1993; Stoneman & Brody, 1993), each sibling's personality may set a chain of transactions within a dyad and thus, contribute to the quality of their relationship. However, the association between neuroticism and characteristics of sibling relationships does not necessarily convey into peer relationships.

Indeed, previously reviewed studies found little evidence of individual differences in sibling interactions carrying over into peer interactions (Harris, 1998).

CONCLUSION

Neuroticism can be observed, defined and reliably measured in children at least from age 3 onwards. The robust trait and its specific constituents are relatively stable over early childhood and across contexts, and foreshadow significant developmental outcomes, particularly in social domains of child development. In sum, different analyses of continuity and change suggest consistency over change for neuroticism, its marker traits, and negative affect over early childhood. This is supported by strong interrater agreement (especially within the same context), moderate to high rank-order temporal stability, small mean-level change, and high individual-level consistency from child age 3 through 6. However, our findings do not preclude a meaningful change in neuroticism within this developmental period: The rank-order stability over time and across contexts (informants) is not perfect, a small percentage of individual children change reliably in neuroticism or related specific traits over time, and there are notable differences in child personality ratings across the informants interacting with the target children in different contexts. The pattern of continuity and change in neuroticism, its constituents, and negative affect over early childhood may be explained by the cumulative continuity (rank-order consistency tends to increase over time), maturity (significant, though small age-related decrease in neuroticism), plasticity (traits can be influenced by environments at any age), and role continuity (consistent roles contribute to continuity of personality) principles of personality development (Roberts et al., 2008).

Along with other reports linking the ICID ratings with child and adolescent social adjustment (Halverson et al., 2003; Slobodskaya, 2007; Slobodskaya & Akhmetova, 2010), our findings (Kavčič et al., 2012; Zupančič & Kavčič, 2007, 2009, 2011; Zupančič et al., 2012) extend previously documented relations between early individual differences in neuroticism and adaptation, most evidently internalizing behavior/problems (e.g., Asendorpf & Van Aken, 2003; De Pauw et al., 2009; Shiner, 2006). Despite several seemingly unfavorable outcomes of early neuroticism, it is important to recognize that it also protects children against the development of externalizing difficulties. Forthcoming investigation may reveal which of the constituents of neuroticism contribute to developmental outcomes and whether there is any substantial increment in the amount of variance predicted by specific traits when compared to the robust trait.

Several forms of person–environment transactions, through which early child personality consistency is maintained and elaborated over time, were proposed (Caspi, 2000; Caspi & Silva, 1995; Roberts & DelVecchio, 2000) and require further empirical inquiry: Evocative (trait expression evokes certain responses in the environment), reactive (different children exposed to the same environment experience it, interpret it and respond to it differently), proactive (children select experiences that best fit their own personality propensities), and manipulative (children attempt to create the environment to suit their personality). Rubin et al. (1999), for example, demonstrated that early childhood shyness contributes to overprotective parenting two years later rather than the other way around, and similar relations were found between early child neuroticism and adjustment to school (Zupančič et al., 2012). However, much less is known about the transactions between early child personality and out-of-home than home environmental influences. Peer groups were proposed to be powerful socialization agents affecting child personality already in early childhood (Harris, 1998), which still awaits substantiation.

Current areas of research, as summarized by Shiner (2006), involve research on genetic as well as intra-individual factors promoting personality continuity/change and contributing to relations between personality and later developmental outcomes. More studies investigating the links between personality and adaptation are also needed to enrich our understanding of the factors that mediate and/or moderate the links between childhood neuroticism and important life outcomes. As shown by Findlay et al. (2009) with school-aged children/adolescent shyness, child coping strategies may be important factors mediating the effect of early neuroticism (and its constituents) on internalizing difficulties. Likewise, other intra-individual child characteristics may moderate the influence of early neuroticism on later developmental outcomes. Asendorpf (1994), for instance, suggested that more intelligent children better handle behavioral inhibition or shyness than their less intelligent peers, and temperament research presented ways in which temperament moderates and is moderated by environmental influences in the prediction of outcomes (see Rothbart & Putnam, 2002).

The FFM traits in young children are just starting to gain research attention and they have received little behaviorally-based empirical validation. Consistently, our findings presented in this chapter are limited to questionnaire data. An extension of questionnaire research on early child neuroticism to observation of its behavioral expressions (see Markey et al., 2004 for measurement of traits in school-aged children) would enhance our understanding of child personality development. As there are probable genetic constraints on the personality traits (including neuroticism; see Shiner, 2006) that can be cultivated in children, future research would certainly benefit from addressing the processes through which adaptive developmental outcomes can be attained in children with widely varied tendencies toward neuroticism.

REFERENCES

Abe, J. A., & Izard, C. E. (1999). A longitudinal study of emotion expression and personality relations in early development. *Journal of Personality and Social Psychology, 77*, 566–577.

Ahadi, S. A., & Rothbart, M. K. (1994). Temperament, development, and the Big Five. In C. F. Halverson, Jr., G. A. Kohnstamm & R. P. Martin (Eds.), *The developing structure of temperament and personality from infancy to adulthood* (pp. 189–208). Hillsdale, NJ: Lawrence Erlbaum Associates.

Ainsworth, M. D. S., Blehar, M. D., Waters, E., & Wall, S. (1978). *Patterns of attachment: A psychological study of the strange situation*. Hillsdale, NJ: Erlbaum.

Angleitner, A., Kohnstamm, G. A., Slotboom, A-. M., & Besevegis, E. (1988). Emotional stability: Developmental perspectives from childhood to adulthood. In G. A. Kohnstamm, C. F. Halverson, Jr., I. Mervielde, & Havill, V. L. (Eds.), *Parental descriptions of child personality. Developmental antecedents of the Big Five* (pp. 85–103). Mahwah, NJ: Lawrence Erlbaum Associates, Publishers.

Asendorpf, J. B. (1994). The malleability of behavior inhibition; A study of individual developmental functions. *Developmental Psychology, 30*, 912–919.

Asendorpf, J.B., & Denissen, J. J. (2006). Predictive validity of personality types versus personality dimensions from early childhood to adulthood: Implications for the distinction between core and surface traits. *Merrill-Palmer Quarterly, 52*, 486–513.

Asendorpf, J. B., & Van Aken, M A. G. (2003). Validity of the Big Five personality judgements in childhood: A 9 year longitudinal study. *European Journal of Personality, 17*, 1–17.

Barbaranelli, C., Caprara, G. V., Rabasca, A., & Pastorelli, C. (2003). A questionnaire for measuring the Big Five in late childhood. *Personality and Individual Differences, 34*, 645–664.

Bishop, G., Spence, S. H., & Mcdonald, C. (2003). Can parents and teachers provide a reliable and valid report of behavioral inhibition? *Child Development, 74*, 1899–1917.

Block, J. H., & Block, J. (1980). The role in ego-control and ego-resiliency in the organization of behavior. In W. A. Collins (Ed.), *Minnesota Symposium on Child Psychology, Vol. 13* (pp. 39–101). Hillsdale, NJ: Erlbaum.

Bradley, R.H., Corwyn, R.F., Burchinal, M., Pipes McAdoo, H., & Garcia Coll, C. (2001). The home environments of children in the United States part II: Relations with behavioral development through age thirteen. *Child Development, 72*, 1868–1886.

Buss, A. H., & Plomin, R. (1984). *Temperament: Early developing personality traits*. Hillsdale, NJ: Lawrence Erlbaum Associates.

Caspi, A. (2000). The child is a father of the man: Personality continuities from childhood to adulthood. *Journal of Personality and Social Psychology, 78*, 158–172.

Caspi, A., Henry, B., McGee, R. O., Moffitt, T. O., & Silva, P. A. (1995). Temperamental origins of child and adolescent behavior problems: From age three to age fifteen. *Child Development, 66*, 55–68.

Caspi, A., Roberts, B. W., & Shiner, R. L. (2005). Personality development: Stability and change. *Annual Review of Psychology, 56*, 453–484.

Caspi, A., & Shiner, R. L (2006). Personality development. In W. Damon, R. Lerner, & N. Eisenberg (Eds.), *Handbook of child psychology: Vol. 3. Social, emotional, and personality development* (pp. 300–364). New York: Wiley.

Caspi, A., & Silva, P. A. (1995). Temperamental qualities at age three predict personality traits in young adulthood: Longitudinal evidence from birth cohort. *Child Development, 66*, 486–498.

De Fruyt, F., Bartels, M., Van Leeuwen, K. G., De Clercq, B., Decuyper, M., & Mervielde, I. (2006). Five types of personality continuity in childhood and adolescence. *Journal of Personality and Social Psychology, 91*, 538–552.

De Fruyt, F. D., & Vollrath, M. (2003). Inter-parent agreement on higher and lower level traits in two countries: effects of parent and child gender. *Personality and Individual Differences, 35*, 289–301.

De Pauw, S. S. W., & Mervielde, I. (2010). Temperament, personality and developmental psychopathology: A review based on conceptual dimensions underlying childhood traits. *Child Psychiatry and Human Development, 41*, 313–329.

De Pauw, S. S. W., Mervielde, I., & Van Leeuwen, K. G. (2009). How are traits related to problem behavior in preschoolers? Similarities and contrasts between temperament and personality. *Journal of Abnormal Child Psychology, 37*, 309–325.

Digman, J. M. (1963), Principal dimensions of child personality as inferred from teachers' judgements. *Child Development, 34*, 43–60.

Digman, J. M. (1989). Five robust trait dimensions: Development, stability, and utility. *Journal of Personality, 57*, 195–214.

Digman, J. M. & Inouye, J. (1986). Further specification of the five robust factors of personality. *Journal of Personality and Social Psychology, 50*, 116–123.

Digman, J. M. in Shmelyov, A. G. (1996). The structure of temperament and personality in Russian children. *Journal of Personality and Social Psychology, 71*, 341–351.

Dunn, J. (1993). *Young children's close relationships: Beyond attachment.* Sage Publications, Inc.

Else-Quest, N. M., Hyde, J. S., Goldsmith, H. H., & Van Hulle, C. A. (2006). Gender differences in temperament: A meta-analysis. *Psychological Bulletin, 132*, 33–72.

Eysenck, S. B. G. (1965). *Manual for the Junior Eysenck Personality Inventory*. London: Hodder & Stoughton.

Eysenck, S. G. B. & Eysenck, H. J. (1980). Impulsiveness and venturesomeness in children. *Personality and Individual Differences*, 1, 73–78.

Feingold, A. (1994). Gender differences in personality: A meta-analysis. *Psychological Bulletin, 116*, 429–456.

Findlay, L. C., Coplan, R. J., & Bowker, A. (2009). Keeping it inside: Shyness, internalizing coping strategies and socio-emotional adjustment in middle childhood. *International Journal of Behavioral Development, 33*, 47–54.

Funder, D. C. (2001). *The personality puzzle*. New York: Norton.

Gallagher, K. C. (2002). Does child temperament moderate the influence of parenting on adjustment? *Developmental Review, 22*, 623–643.

Gomes, L., & Livesey, D. (2008). Exploring the link between impulsivity and peer relations in 5- and 6-year-old children. *Child: Care, Health and Development, 34,* 763–770.

Graziano, W. G., Jensen-Campbell, & Sullivan-Logan (1998). Temperament, activity, and expectations for later personality development. *Journal of Personality and Social Psychology, 74*, 1266–1277.

Grist, C. L., & McCord, D. M. (2010). Individual differences in preschool children: Temperament or personality? *Infant and Child Development, 19*, 264–274.

Hagekull, B. (1994). Infant temperament and early childhood functioning: Possible relations to the five-factor model. In C. F. Halverson Jr., G. A. Kohnstamm & R. P. Martin (Eds.), *The developing structure of temperament and personality from infancy to adulthood* (pp. 227–240). Hillsdale, NJ: Lawrence Erlbaum Associates.

Halverson, C. F. (2003). *Culture, age, and personality development.* Paper presented at the 11th European Conference on Developmental Psychology, Milan, Italy.

Halverson, C. F., Havill, V. L., Deal, J., Baker, S. R., Victor J. B., Pavlopoulos, V., Besevegis, E., & Wen, L. (2003). Personality structure as derived from parental ratings of free descriptions of children: The Inventory of Child Individual Differences. *Journal of Personality*, *71*(6), 995–1026.

Harris, J.R. (1998). *The nurture assumption: Why children turn out the way they do.* New York, London, Toronto, Sydney: The Free Press.

Havill, V. L., Allen, K., Halverson, C. F., Jr., & Kohnstamm, G. A. (1994). Parents' use of the Big Five categories in their natural language descriptions of children. In C. F. Halverson, Jr., G. A. Kohnstamm & R. P. Martin (Eds.), *The developing structure of temperament and personality from infancy to adulthood* (pp. 371–386). Hillsdale, NJ: Lawrence Erlbaum Associates.

Izard, C. E., Dougherty, L. M., & Hembree, E. A. (1983). *A system for identifying affect expression by holistic judgements (AFFEX).* Newark: University of Delaware, Computer Network Services and University Media Services.

Jacobson, N. S., & Truax, P. (1991). Clinical significance: A statistical approach to defining meaningful change in psychotherapy research. *Journal of Consulting and Clinical Psychology, 59*(1), 12–19.

John, O. P., Caspi, A., Robins, R. W., Moffitt, T. E., & Stouthamer-Loeber, M. (1994). The "Little Five": Exploring the nomological network of the Five-

Factor Model of personality in adolescent boys. *Child Development, 65*, 160–178.

Kavčič, T., Podlesek, A., & Zupančič, M. (2012). The role of early childhood personality in developmental course of social adjustment. *International Journal of Behavioral Development, 36*, 215–225.

Kavčič, T., & Zupančič, M. (2006). *Osebnost otrok in njihovi medsebojni odnosi v družini [Children's personality and their interpersonal relationships within the family]*. Ljubljana: ZIFF.

Kavčič, T., & Zupančič, M. (2011). Sibling relationship and personality in early/middle childhood from parent's perception. *Contemporary Psychology, 14*, 119–133.

Knyazev, G. G., Zupančič, M., & Slobodskaya, H. R. (2008). Child personality in Slovenia and Russia: Structure and mean level of traits in parent and self-ratings. *Journal of Cross Cultural Psychology, 39*(3), 317–334.

Kochanska, G. (1997). Multiple pathways to conscience for children with different temperaments: From toddlerhood to age five. *Developmental Psychology, 33*, 228–240.

Kohnstamm, G. A., Halverson, C. F., Mervielde, I., & Havill, V. L. (Eds.) (1998). *Parental descriptions of child personality: Developmental antecedents of the Big Five*. Mahwah, NJ: Lawrence Erlbaum.

LaFreniere, P. J., Dumas, J. E., Zupančič, M., Gril, A., & Kavčič, T. (2001). *Vprašalnik o socialnem vedenju. Priročnik* [Social Competence and Behavior Evaluation Scale. Manual]. Ljubljana: Center for Psychodiagnostic Resources.

Laidra, K., Pullman, H., & Allik, J. (2007). Personality and intelligence as predictors of academic achievement: A cross-sectional study from elementary to secondary school. *Personality and Individual Differences, 42*(3), 441–451.

Lamb, M. E., Chuang, S. S., Wessels, H., Broberg, A. G., & Hwang, C. P. (2002). Emergence and construction validation of the Big Five factors in early childhood: A longitudinal analysis of their ontogeny in Sweden. *Child Development, 73*, 1517–1524.

Little, T. D., & Wanner, B. (1998). *Validity of a Big-Five Personality Inventory for Children (B5P-C)*. Contribution presented at the Biennial Meeting of the International Society for Behavioral Development, Bern, Switzerland.

Lynn, R., & Martin, T. (1997). Gender differences in extraversion, neuroticism, and psychoticism in 37 nations. *Journal of Social Psychology, 137*, 369–373.

Markey, C. N., Markey, P. M., Ericksen, A. J., & Tinsey, B. J. (2002). A preliminary validation of preadolescents' self-reports using the Five-Factor Model of personality. *Journal of Research in Personality, 36*(2), 173–181.

Markey, P. M., Markey, C. N., & Tinsley, B. J. (2004). Children's behavioral manifestations of the Five-Factor Model of personality. *Personality and Social Psychology Bulletin, 30,* 423–432.

McCrae, R. R., & Costa, P. T., Jr. (1997). Personality trait structure as a human universal. *American Psychologist, 52*, 509–516.

McCrae, R. R., & Costa, P. T. Jr. (2003). *Personality in adulthood: A Five-Factor Theory perspective* (2nd ed.). New York: Guilford.

McCrae, R. R., Costa, P. T. Jr., Ostendorf, F., Angleitner, A., Hrebičkova, M., Avia, M. D. et al. (2000). Nature over nature: Temperament, personality, and the life span development. *Journal of Personality and Social Psychology, 78*, 173–186.

McCrae, R. R., Terracianno, A., & 78 members of the Personality Profiles of Cultures Project (2005). Universal features of personality traits from the observer's perspective: Data from 50 cultures. *Journal of Personality and Social Psychology*, *88*, 547–561.

Measelle, J. R., John, O. P., Ablow, J. C., Cowan, P. A., & Cowan, C. P. (2005). Can children provide coherent, stable, and valid self-reports on the Big Five dimensions? A longitudinal study from ages 5 to 7. *Journal of Personality and Social Psychology,89*, 90–106.

Mervielde, I., Buyst, V., & De Fruyt, F. (1995). The validity of the Big-Five as a model for teacher's ratings of individual differences among children aged 4–12 years. *Personality and Individual Differences*, *18*(4), 525–534.

Mervielde, I., & De Fruyt, F. (2002). Assessing children's traits with the Hierarchical Personality Inventory for Children (HiPIC). In B. De Raad, & M. Perugini (Eds.), *Big Five assessment* (pp. 129–146). Gottingen: Hogrefe & Hoger Publishers.

Miller, S. R., Tserakhava, V., & Miller, C. J. (2011). ''My child is shy and has no friends: What does parenting have to do with it?'' *Journal of Youth and Adolescence, 40*, 442–452. doi:10.1007/s10964-010-9550-5

Prinzie, P., & Deković, M. (2008). Continuity and change of childhood personality characteristics through the lens of teachers. *Personality and Individual Differences, 45*, 82–88.

Puklek, M., & Gril, A. (1999). Socioemocionalne in vedenjske značilnosti otrok ob vstopu v solo [Socio-emotional and behavioral characteristics of children starting school]. In M. Zupančič (Ed.), *Razvojnopsihološke značilnosti različno starih otrok ob vstopu v solo [Psychological characteristics of children starting school at different ages]* (pp. 43–66). Ljubljana: i2.

Roberts, B. W., Caspi, A., & Moffitt, T. E. (2001). The kids are alright: Growth and stability in personality development from adolescence to adulthood. *Journal of Personality and Social Psychology, 81*, 670–683.

Roberts, B. W., & Del Vecchio, W. F. (2000). The rank-order consistency of personality traits from childhood to old age: A quantitative review of longitudinal studies. *Psychological Bulletin, 126,* 3–25.

Roberts, B. W., Wood, D., & Caspi, A. (2008). The development of personality traits in adulthood. In O. P. John, R. W. Robins & L. A. Pervin (Eds.), *Handbook of personality: Theory and research* (pp. 375–398). New York: Guilford Press.

Robins, R. W., Fraley, R. C., Roberts, B. W. in Trzesniewski, K. H. (2001). A longitudinal study of personality change in young adulthood. *Journal of Personality, 69*, 617–640.

Rothbart, M. K. (1981). Measurement of temperament in infancy. *Child Development, 52*, 569–578.

Rothbart, M. K. (2007). Temperament, development, and personality. *Current Directions in Psychological Science, 16*, 207–212.

Rothbart, M. K., Ahadi, S. A., Hershey, K. L., & Fisher, P. (2001). Investigations of temperament at three to seven years: The Children's Behavior Questionnaire. *Child Development, 72*, 1394–1408.

Rothbart, M. K., & Bates, J. E. (1998). Temperament. In W. Damon (Series Ed.) & N. Eisenberg (Vol. Ed.), *Handbook of child psychology: Vol. 3. Social, emotional, and personality development* (pp. 105–176). New York: Wiley.

Rothbart, M. K., & Derryberry, D. (2002). Temperament in children. In C. von Hofsten & L. Backman (Eds.), *Psychology at the turn of the millennium: Vol. 2. Social, developmental,and clinical perspectives* (pp. 17–35). New York: Taylor & Francis.

Rothbart, M. K., Posner, M. I., & Hershey, K. L. (1995). Temperament, attention, and psychopathology. In D. Cicchetti & D. J. Cohen (Eds.), *Developmental psychopathology: Vol. 1, Theory and methods* (pp. 315–342). New York: Wiley.

Rothbart, M. K. & Putnam, S. P. (2002). Temperament and socialization. In L. Pulkkinen & A. Caspi (Eds.), *Paths to successful development. Personality in the life course* (pp.19–45). Cambridge, UK Cambridge University Press.

Rubin, K. H., Nelson, L. J., Hastings, O., & Asendorpf, J. (1999). The transaction between parents' perceptions of their children's shyness and their parenting styles. *International Journal of Behavioral Development, 23*(4), 937–958.

Shiner, R. L. (2005). A developmental perspective on personality disorders: Lessons from research on normal personality development in childhood and adolescence. *Journal of Personality Disorders, 19*, 202–210.

Shiner, R. L. (2006). Temperament and personality in childhood. In D. K. Mroczek in T. D. Little (Eds.), *Handbook of personality development* (pp. 213–230). Mahwah, NJ: Lawrence Erlbaum Associates Publishers.

Silva, P. A., & Stanton, W. (Eds.) (1996). *From child to adult: The Dunedin study*. Oxford, UK: Oxford University Press.

Slobodskaya, H. R. (2005). *Personality as predictor of behavioural and emotional problems in Russian children of different ages*. Contribution presented at 12th European Conference on Developmental Psychology, La Laguna, Spain.

Slobodskaya, H. R. (2007). The associations among the Big Five, Behavioural Inhibition and Behavioural Approach systems and child and adolescent adjustment in Russia. *Personality and Individual Differences*, *43*, 913–924.

Slobodskaya, H. R., & Akhmetova, O. A. (2010). Personality development and problem behavior in Russian children and adolescents. *International Journal of Behavioral Development, 34,* 441–451.

Slotboom, A-. M., Havill, V. L., Pavlopoulos, V., & De Fruyt, F. (1998). Developmental changes in personality descriptions of children: A cross-national comparison of parental descriptions of children. In G. A. Kohnstamm, C. F. Halverson, Jr., I. Mervielde, & Havill, V. L. (Eds.), *Parental descriptions of child personality. Developmental antecedents of the Big Five* (pp. 127–153). Mahwah, NJ: Lawrence Erlbaum Associates, Publishers.

Stoneman, Z., & Brody, G. H. (1993). Sibling temperaments, conflict, warmth, and role asymmetry. *Child Development, 64*, 1786–1800.

Thomas, A., & Chess, S. (1977). *Temperament and development.* New York: Brunner/Mazel.

Thomas, A., & Chess, S. (1982). Temperament and follow-up to adulthood. In R. Porter & G. M. Collins (Eds.), *Temperamental differences in infants and young children* (pp. 168–175). London: Pitman.

Thomas, A., Chess, S., Birch, H., Hertzig, M., & Korn, S. (1963). *Behavioral individuality in early childhood.* New York: New York University Press.

Van Leeuwen, K. G., Mervielde, I., Braet, C., & Bosmans, G. (2004). Child personality and parental behavior as moderators of problem behavior: Variable- and person-centered approaches. *Developmental Psychology, 40*(6), 1028–1046.

Van Lieshout, C. F. M., & Haselager, G. J. T. (1994). The Big Five personality factots in Q-sort descriptions of children and adolescents. In C. F. Halverson Jr., G. A. Kohnstamm & R. P. Martin (Eds.), *The developing structure of temperament and personality from infancy to adulthood* (pp. 293–318). Hillsdale, NJ: Lawrence Erlbaum Associates.

Zahra, D., & Hedge, C. (2010). The reliable change index: Why isn't it more popular in academic psychology. *Psychology Postgraduate Affairs Group Quarterly, 76*, 14–19.

Zupančič, M. (2001). Parental free descriptions of their infants/toddlers: Do they resemble the Five-Factor Model of personality? *Horizons of Psychology, 10*(3), 21–42.

Zupančič, M. (2004). Parental free descriptions of child personality: Applicability of the five-factor model taxonomy from infancy through pre-school years. *Studia Psychologica,46,* 145–162.

Zupančič, M., Gril, A. in Kavčič, T. (2006). Child and adolescent personality: Its structure, age trends and gender differences. *Studia Psychologica*, *48*, 311–332.

Zupančič, M., & Kavčič, T. (2002). Toddler's and pre-school children's characteristics as perceived by mothers and pre-school teachers: Do their free descriptions resemble the five-factor model of personality? *Horizons of Psychology, 11*(1), 7–24.

Zupančič, M., & Kavčič, T. (2004). Personality structure in Slovenian three-year-olds: The Inventory of Child Individual Differences. *Horizons of Psychology*, *13*(1), 9–27.

Zupančič, M., & Kavčič, T. (2005). Gender differences in personality through early childhood: A multiple-informant perspective. *Horizons of Psychology, 14*(2), 11–38.

Zupančič, M. in Kavčič, T. (2007). *Otroci od vrtca do šole: razvoj osebnosti in socialnega vedenja ter učna uspešnost prvošolcev* [*Children from preschool to school: Development of personality and social behavior, and academic achievement in the first grade*]. Ljubljana: Znanstvenoraziskovalni inštitut Filozofske fakultete.

Zupančič, M., & Kavčič, T. (2009). *Vprašalnik o medosebnih razlikah pri otrocih in mladostnikih (VMR-OM): priročnik [The Inventory of Child and Adolescent Individual Differences (ICID): The Manual]*. Ljubljana: Center for Psychodiagnostic Resources.

Zupančič, M., & Kavčič, T. (2011). Factors of social adjustment to school: Child's personality, family and pre-school. *Early Child Development and Care, 181*, 493–504.

Zupančič, M., Podlesek, A., & Kavčič, T. (July, 2012). *The transaction between teachers' perceptions of child personality and social adjustment in (pre)school.* Contribution presented at the 16th European Conference on Personality, Trieste, Italy.

Zupančič, M., Slobodskaya, H. R., & Knyazev, G. G. (2008). Gender differences in child/adolescent personality traits. *Horizons of Psychology, 17*(3), 43–61.

Zupančič, M., Sočan, G., & Kavčič, T. (2009). Consistency in adult reports on child personality over the pre-school years. *European Journal of Developmental Psychology*, *6*(4), 455–480.

In: Psychology of Neuroticism
Editor: Kristel Parn
ISBN: 978-1-62808-150-3

Chapter 2

THE RELATIONS BETWEEN THE PERCEIVED PARENTING STYLES AND THE NEUROTICISM IN CHILDREN AND ADOLESCENTS

Belén Mesurado[1,2,*]
and María Cristina Richaud de Minzi[1,2]
[1]Interdisciplinary Center of Mathematical and Experimental Psychology Research, Buenos Aires, Argentina
[2]National Council of Scientific and Technological Research (CONICET), Buenos Aires, Argentina

ABSTRACT

The objectives of this chapter are: 1). To study differences, according to gender and age, in the perception of the father and mother parental styles (acceptance, pathological control and extreme autonomy) in childhood and adolescence; 2). To study differences in neuroticism dimensions (self-criticism, vulnerability, anxiety, perceived lack of competence), according to gender and age; 3). To study the relationship of parental styles as perceived by children with neuroticism according to gender and ages. The total sample consisted of 1494 Argentinean children and adolescents. It included 517 middle-class children aged 8-11 (M = 10.26, SD = .88), both genders (253 boys and 264 girls), and 977

[*] Corresponding author: Belén Mesurado. Tte. Gral. Perón 2158, 1040 Buenos Aires, Argentina. E-mail: bmesurado@conicet.gov.ar.

adolescents aged 12-16 (M = 12.85, SD = .86) both genders (431 boys and 546 girls), from primary and high schools in Buenos Aires and Tucumán, Argentina. The results indicate that father and mother parental style are perceived in a different way by children, according to gender and ages. On the other hand, the results of this study revealed statistically significant differences in neuroticism dimensions, with female children showing higher levels of neuroticism, especially self-criticism, vulnerability and perceived lack of competence, the results shown that children who show demonstrate higher levels of self-criticism, vulnerability and anxiety than adolescents. Lastly, we found that the only parenting dimension that is associated with neuroticism is pathological control, that is, excessive, intrusive control, based on guilt, which implies the implementation of strict norms, punishments and scolding, based on a negative evaluation of the child and distancing through rejection.

NEUROTICISM TRAIT

Neuroticism is an important personality, characterized by anxiety, moodiness, worry, envy and jealousy. Most theoretical models of personality include the dimension of neuroticism (Eysenck, 1967, Reynaud, El Khoury-Malhame, Rossier, Blin, and Khalfa, 2012) that is a complex construct that includes several different traits and facets, such as a tendency to be worried and anxious (Canli et al., 2001), to be emotionally unstable (Naquin and Holton, 2002; Judge and Ilies, 2002), to experience negative feelings (Larsen and Ketelaar, 1991; Robinson, Ode, Moeller, and Goetz, 2007), and denotes an increased general proneness to negative emotional reactivity and arousal. Neuroticism is one of the four dimensions that encompass core self-evaluations, one's basic appraisal of oneself, along with locus, self-efficacy, and self-esteem (Judge, Locke, and Durham, 1997).

Neuroticism and psychological distress are related but distinct constructs; neuroticism is considered to be a stable and relatively enduring trait, with a strong genetic component (Krueger, Caspi, and Moffitt, 2000), representing a tendency to experience distress frequently (Goldberg, 2001; McCrae, et. al., 2002;Van Os and Jones, 1999).

In fact, subjects with high neuroticism scores are more distressed by negative mood induction than those with low scores and they tend to be more psychologically reactive to stressors (Larsen and Ketelaar, 1989, 1991).

Lahey (2009) argues that the personality trait of neuroticism refers to a relatively stable tendency to respond with negative emotions to threat, frustration, or loss. The greater one's neuroticism, the more threat will be perceived in a variety of situations (Craske, 1999). In this perspective, subjects high in neuroticism are vulnerable to stress. A high neuroticism score is a predictor of the vulnerability to develop depression and is related to a life time prevalence of depression (Hansenne, et. al. 1999; Stewart, Ebmeier, and Deary, 2005). People high in neuroticism experience negative affects in response to challenges and view themselves and the surrounding world negatively (Bruck and Allen, 2003).

Neuroticism and extraversion traits -being extraversion a tendency to be gregarious, assertive, to seek excitement and challenges (see Costa and McCrae, 1991)- may affect overall self-rated health or subjective wellbeing. In this sense, Costa and McCrae (1980) reported that individuals with higher scores on extraversion and those with lower scores on neuroticism showed greater happiness, and Chico Librán (2006) showed that the neuroticism trait rather than the extraversion trait was more strongly, inversely associated with subjective wellbeing, as measured by satisfaction with life and other aspects. Neuroticism is also supposed to have a negative impact on wellbeing within the family (Schneewind and Kupsch, 2007).

Finally evidence is found about a detrimental effect of high neuroticism on relationship quality and on the perception of availability of social support (Swickert and Owens, 2010). Several studies have presented neuroticism as related to dissatisfaction in relationships with peers and family of origin (Belsky, Jaffee, Caspi, Moffitt, and Silva, 2003; Neyer and Asendorpf, 2001).

Parental Styles

Several recent studies have indicated that during childhood there is a relationship between various forms of psychological disturbances and perceived parenting style (Wolfradt, Hempel, and Miles, 2003). Darling and Steinberg (1993) have defined parenting style "as a constellation of attitudes toward the child that is communicated to the child and that, taken together, create an emotional climate in which the parents' behaviours are expressed" (p. 488).

Researchers have identified three central dimensions of parenting as a means for explaining substantial variations in how parenting is measured (Skinner, Johnson, and Snyder, 2005).

These dimensions of the parent-child relationship are associated with individual differences in development during childhood and used with greatest consistency and analytical strength. They are (a) warmth versus rejection, (b) behavioural control versus chaos, and (c) autonomy support versus coercion.

The warmth dimension considers whether, "parents intentionally foster individuality, self-regulation, and self-assertion by being attuned, supportive, and acquiescent to the child's special needs and demands" (Baumrind, 1991, p. 62). Warmth relationship is crucial for attaining positive developmental outcomes, such as self-mastery, emotional regulation, and interpersonal closeness (Bugental and Grusec, 2006), while at the other end of the spectrum, lack of responsiveness may be associated with behavioural problems (Rothbaum and Weisz, 1994). On the other hand, the behavioural control refers "to the claims parents make on the child to become integrated into the family whole by their maturity demands, supervision, disciplinary efforts, and willingness to confront the child who disobeys" (Baumrind, 1991, pp. 61–62).

There is much evidence (Mesurado and Richaud, 2013; Richaud de Minzi, 2006a, 2010; Richaud, Lemos, and Mesurado, 2011; Samper, et al., 2006) that parental styles are important factors in children's cognitive, emotional and social development. Parenting styles perceived to be authoritarian and controlling are closely related to psychological disturbances in childhood, while lack of discipline or lack of responsiveness (e.g. no control, no punishment) is related to poor psychological adjustment (Johnson, Shulman, and Collins, 1991).

Spinath and O'Connor (2003) showed, working with non-clinical samples, that elevated Neuroticism has been associated with self-reported parental rejection by children. Evidence was found that when parents exert pathological control over their children, meaning excessive control with low levels of displays of affection and acceptance, children develop higher levels of neuroticism.

While, when children perceive that their parents accept them, they report lower levels of neuroticism (Mesurado and Richaud de Minzi, in press). However, this study did not show whether these relationships between perceived parental styles and children's personality traits are maintained throughout adolescence.

Though parents are identified as one of the most significant influences on cognitive, emotional and social development during childhood and adolescence (Belsky, 1990; Burbach and Borduin, 1986; Maccoby and Martin, 1983), few studies have focused on studying the influence of parental styles on children's personalities during mid-to-late childhood and early adolescence.

It is essential to keep in mind that boys and girls perceive parental styles differently according to gender and ages (Mestre, Samper, Tur, and Díez,

2001). Girls are expected to be more nurturing and concerned with the social judgement of others, while boys are expected to be more autonomous. Consequently, stereotypical gender socialization leads to a lower sense of self-mastery and control and a higher concern for external evaluation in girls than in boys (Blehar and Oren, 1999; Ruble, Greulich, Pomerantz, and Gochberg, 1993). Several studies demonstrate important differences in personality traits according to gender and ages (McCrae, et al., 2004; Weisberg, DeYoung, and Hirsh, 2011). In fact, it is well acknowledged that personality traits may develop differently in males and females not only because of gender-based social experiences (Srivastava, John, Gosling, and Potter, 2003) but because biological differences (Shaffer, 2009). Moreover levels of personality traits changes with development (Costa Jr., and McCrae, 2006; Roberts, Walton, and Viechtbauer, 2005).

In line with what it was expressed above, the objectives of this chapter are:

1 To study differences, according to gender and age, in the perception of the paternal and maternal parenting styles (acceptance, pathological control and extreme autonomy) in childhood and adolescence;
2 To study differences in neuroticism dimensions (self-criticism, vulnerability, anxiety, perceived lack of Competence), according to gender and age;
3 To study the relationship of parenting styles as perceived by children with neuroticism according to gender and ages.

METHODS

Participants and Procedure

The total sample consisted of 1494 Argentinean children and adolescents. It included 517 middle-class children aged 8-11 (M = 10.26, SD = .88), both genders (253 boys and 264 girls), and 977 adolescents aged 12-16 (M = 12.85, SD = .86) both genders (431 boys and 546 girls), from primary and high schools in Buenos Aires and Tucumán, Argentina. The participants completed the questionnaires in groups of approximately 20 children in one session of 30 minutes.

Ethical Procedures

Consent for this project was obtained at multiple levels. First, heads of schools at potential research sites were asked to discuss the project with the researchers. They were provided with a copy of the research proposal, and the characteristics of the research were explained.

Once permission was received from heads of schools, a letter was sent to the household of each child explaining the aims of the project and the procedures to evaluate children. They were clearly told that participation was voluntary and anonymous. Written permission from each father and mother was obtained before data collection began. Finally, children were informed of the purpose of the study. They were then instructed on data collection procedures, and reminded that they could refuse to answer questions if they chose to. There were no objections from the children.

Instruments

1. Children's Perception of Parental Relationships

The Argentine Scale of Children's Perception of their Relationships with their Parents (Richaud de Minzi, 2007) is a self-report questionnaire designed to be used to assess children's perceptions of parent–child relationships. It comprises 32 items. The answer to each item may be Yes, More or less, or No.

Two factor analyses were carried out, one for fathers and one for mothers. The KMO was .95 for mothers and .93 for fathers. The oblimin solution method of principal components was employed. For the definitions of factors only the variables with a factor weight of |.30| or more were taken into account (Norman and Streiner, 1994).

In the two factor analyses the Cattell graphic method was employed for the determination of a number of factors.

The two factor analyses showed five dimensions: Acceptance (seven items; $\alpha = .92$ for mothers, $\alpha = .89$ for fathers), Normal or Acceptable Control (five items; $\alpha = .75$ for both parents), Strict Control, though non-pathological, it is less accepted (5 items; alpha .81 for mothers and alpha .65 for fathers), Pathological Control (10 items; $\alpha = .72$ for mothers, $\alpha = .81$ for fathers) and Negligence (five items, $\alpha = .60$ for both parents).

The first type of relationship includes the following dimensions: acceptance, child centeredness, acceptance of individuation and positive involvement.

The second one includes control-related items, but only those that are correlated with acceptance (For example, “They make sure I come back home on time”). The third one, strict control, includes items such as: “He/she insists I should do my homework,” or “He/she makes sure I obey his/her orders.” The fourth type, pathological control, covers the following dimensions: hostile control (“They believe they punishing me they will mend my misbehaviour”), instilling persistent anxiety (“When I misbehave, they worry because I will suffer the consequences when I become an adult”), withdrawal of relations (“If I do something wrong they stop talking me”) and control through guilt (“I get the blame for everything they have to do for me”). And the fifth, negligence (“Let me go anyplace I please without asking”).

The correspondence between the Schaeffer (1965) taxonomy with Baumrind’s would be as follows: Acceptance-Responsiveness; Accepted Control—Demandingness; Strict control—High Demandingness; Pathological control—Very High Demandingness; and Extreme Autonomy—Lack of Demandingness. In this work we decided to study the effect of three parental styles: Acceptance, Extreme Autonomy and Pathological Control.

2. Personality Traits

The Argentine Scale of Personality for Children (Lemos, 2006). This instrument was constructed to measure personality traits in children. It is based on the Costa and McCrae NEOPI-R (Costa and McCrae, 1980; McCrae and Costa, 1991; McCrae, et al. 2004; McCrae, Costa Jr, and Martin, 2005; Costa Jr, McCrae, and Martin, 2008) that operationalizes the “Big Five” model of personality. The Argentine Scale of Personality for Children is composed of 46 items.

The answer to each item may be Yes, Sometimes or No. This questionnaire assesses five personality factors: Neuroticism ($\alpha = .79$) (e.g., “I need other people to help me solve my problems no matter how small they are”), Extraversion ($\alpha = .80$) (e.g., “I like being in places with lots of other young people”, “I like scaring movies”), Openness to Experience ($\alpha = .56$) (e.g., “I thinks it’s interesting to learn and develop new hobbies”), Conscientiousness ($\alpha = .71$) (e.g., “I am organized, I like to keep everything in its place”) and Agreeableness ($\alpha = .77$) (e.g., “I can trick someone without them realizing it” -reverse item-).

This research will use the Neuroticism dimension of the Argentina Scale of Personality for Children (Lemos, 2006), which allows for the measurement of four different facets: Self-criticism, Vulnerability, Anxiety and Perceived of Lack Competence.

The Self-criticism facet (made up of four items, e.g. "I feel bad when other person told me that I did anything bad"), it is defined by feelings of embarrassment, sensitiveness to ridicule and feelings of inferiority. Children with high levels of Self-criticism would be more demanding on themselves, they would not let themselves make mistakes, and if they made them, it would affect them quite a lot.

The Vulnerability facet (made up of 2 items, e.g. "I need someone else to help me solve my problems (difficulties) no matter how small they may be") would be associated with mood swings and difficulty controlling negative environmental stresses. The children who score high on this facet would be more likely to feel unable to face environmental demands, which would generally be perceived as excessive.

The Anxiety facet (made up of 3 items, e.g. "Just thinking about having a test at school makes me nervous") being tense, nervous with a visible tendency to worry and experience fear. Last is the Perceived Lack of Competence facet (composed by 5 items, e.g. "I find it hard to learn") refers to the perceived lack of ability to face daily situations.

Statistical Procedure

In order to test our first objective about whether perceived paternal and maternal parental style differ according to gender (male and female) and according to age (children aged 8-11 and adolescents ages 12-16), we conducted two Multivariate Analysis of Variance (MANOVA). Different dimensions of fathers' and mothers' parental style were entered as dependent variables and gender and age as fixed factors.

Another Multivariate Analysis of Variance (MANOVA) was conducted to study whether the four facets neuroticism personality traits differ according to gender (male and female) and according to age (children aged 8-11 and adolescents ages 12-16).

The four facets neuroticism personality traits were entered as dependent variables and gender and age as fixed factors.

Finally, two multiple regressions analyses were conducted to examine relationships between children's perception of parental styles (Acceptance, Pathological Control and Negligence) and Neurotic personality trait, one for males and one for females. The age was used as control variable.

RESULTS

Table 1 displays the descriptive statistics of perception of parental relationship and of facets of neuroticism personality traits according to gender (male and female) and age (children aged 8-11 and adolescents ages 12-16).

Table 1. Descriptive statistics of Perception of Parental Relationship and facets of neuroticism personality traits

Variables	Children				Adolescents			
	Males		Females		Males		Females	
	M	SD	M	SD	M	SD	M	SD
Parental Style Father Acceptance	2.57	.42	2.53	.37	2.47	.47	2.46	.50
Mother Acceptance	2.66	.32	2.68	.32	2.58	.39	2.63	.37
Father Pathological Control	2.09	.42	1.87	.40	1.87	.47	1.73	.46
Mother Pathological Control	2.17	.44	1.94	.40	1.96	.47	1.82	.46
Father Extreme Autonomy	2.05	.54	1.9	.53	1.2	.54	1.82	.54
Mother Extreme Autonomy	1.96	.51	1.87	.46	1.93	.47	1.79	.45
Neuroticism Dimensions								
Self-Criticism	2.36	.48	2.44	.43	2.24	.51	2.37	.45
Vulnerability	2.31	.65	2.45	.63	2.19	.64	2.44	.52
Anxiety	2.35	.40	2.31	.35	2.19	.40	2.2	.34
Perceived Lack of Competence	1.65	.47	1.68	.48	1.67	.50	1.75	.48

Comparison of Fathers' Parental Styles According to Gender and Age

To test our first objective regarding fathers' parental styles according to children gender and age, we conducted a -three (father's acceptance, father's pathological control and father's extreme autonomy) by two (male vs. female) by two (children vs. adolescents)- MANOVA. Results showed significant overall effect in gender, Hotelling's = $F(3, 1472) = 29.55, p \leq .001$ and in age, Hotelling's $F(3, 1472) = 23.94, p \leq .001$.

The analysis of uni-variant contrasts shows significant differences between males and females in father pathological control, $F(1, 1474) = 55.47$, $p \leq .001$, and father extreme autonomy, $F(1, 1474) = 24.63, p \leq .001$, but not in father's acceptance. Boys perceive their fathers to exercise higher levels of extreme autonomy and pathological control than do girls (see Figure, 1).

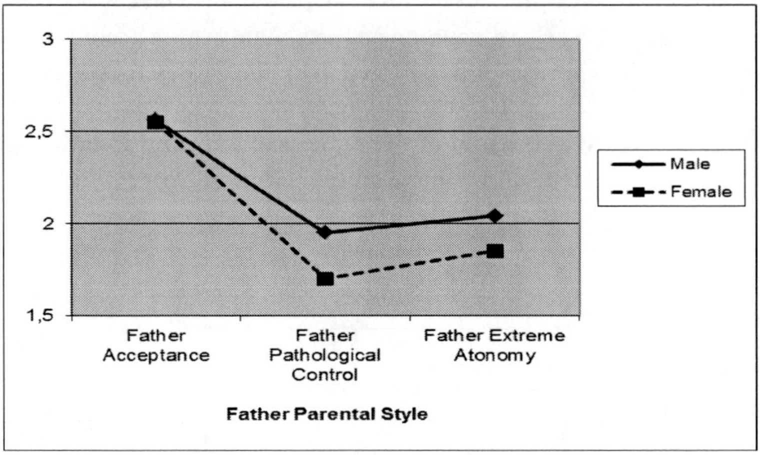

Figure 1. Comparison of fathers' parental styles according to children's gender.

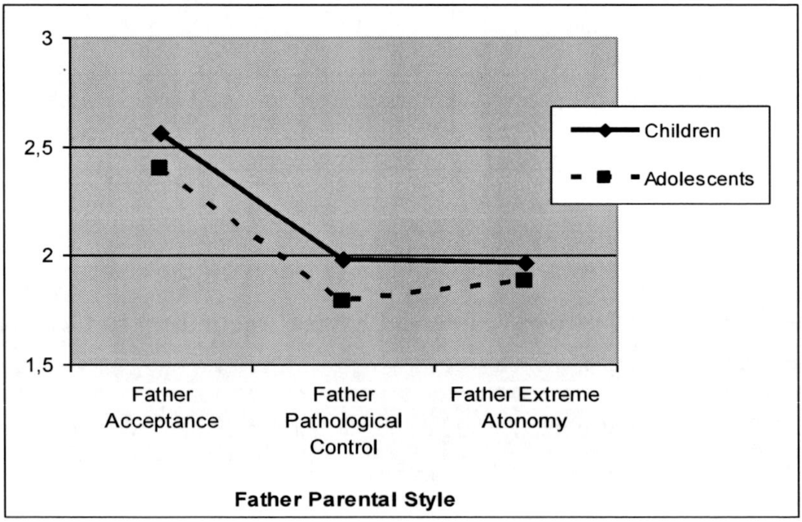

Figure 2. Comparison of fathers' parental styles according to age.

Univariate analyses also revealed significant differences between children and adolescents in father acceptance, $F(1, 1474) = 12.95$, $p \leq .001$; father pathological control, $F(1, 1474) = 55.36$, $p \leq .001$, and father extreme autonomy, $F(1, 1474) = 5.96$, $p \leq .01$. Children perceive their parents to exercise higher levels of pathological control and acceptance than do adolescents. Children also perceive higher levels of extreme autonomy than adolescents although this difference is less pronounced (see Figure, 2).

Comparison of Mothers' Parental Style According to Gender and Age

To test differences in mothers' parental styles according to children gender, we conducted a -three (mother acceptance, mother pathological control and mother extreme autonomy) by two (male vs. female) by two (children vs. adolescents)- MANOVA. Results showed significant overall effect in gender, Hotelling's = $F(3, 1484) = 25.57$, $p \leq .001$ and for ages $F(3, 1484) = 18.31$, $p \leq .001$.

Univariate analyses revealed significant differences according to gender for mother pathological control, $F(1, 1486) = 53.49$, $p \leq .001$, and mother extreme autonomy, $F(1, 1486) = 18.55$, $p \leq .001$, although no significant differences were identified in mother's acceptance. Boys perceive their mothers to exercise higher levels of extreme autonomy and pathological control than do daughters (see Figure, 3).

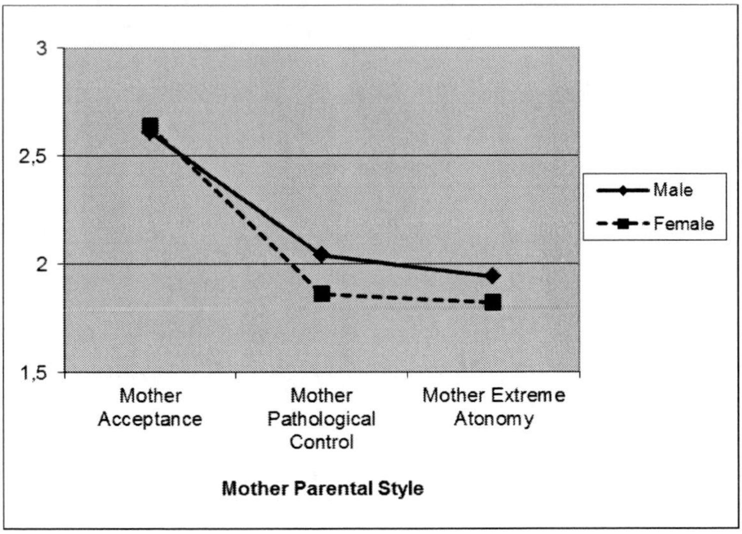

Figure 3. Comparison of mothers' parental styles according to children's gender.

Univariate analyses revealed significant differences between children and adolescents in mother acceptance, $F(1, 1486) = 9.20$, $p \leq .01$, mother pathological control, $F(1, 1486) = 41.28$, $p \leq .001$, and mother extreme autonomy, $F(1, 1486) = 3.84$, $p \leq .05$. The children perceive their mother to exercise higher levels of acceptance, pathological control and extreme autonomy than do adolescents.

However, it is important to underscore the fact that differences in perception between acceptance and extreme autonomy are not very significant among children and adolescents (see Figure 4).

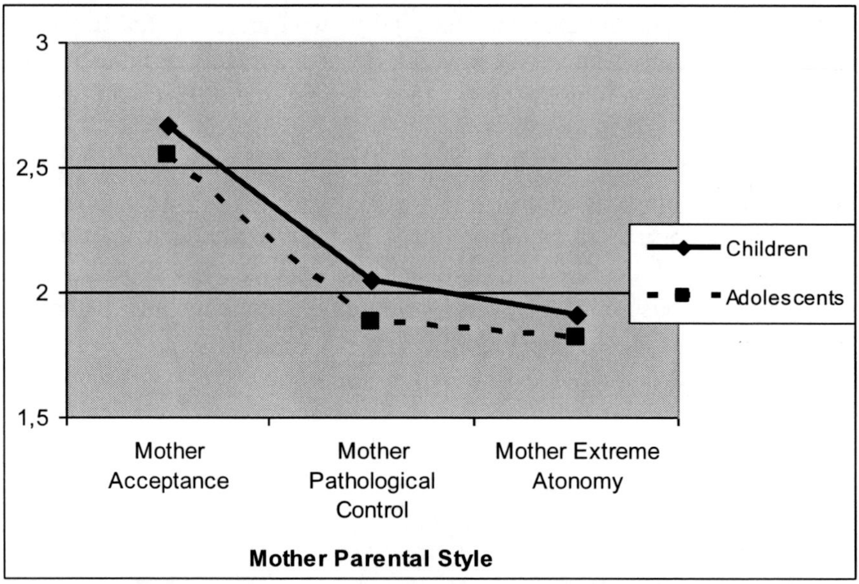

Figure 4. Comparison of mothers' parental styles according to age.

Comparison of the Neuroticism Dimensions (Self-Criticism, Vulnerability, Anxiety, Perceived Lack of Competence) According to Gender and Age

To test our second objective regarding differences in the neuroticism dimensions across gender and age, we conducted a - four (Self-Criticism, Vulnerability, Anxiety, Perceived Lack of Competence) by two (Male vs. Female) by two (children vs. adolescents)- MANOVA. Results indicated significant overall effect in gender, Hotelling's= $F(4, 1483) = 14.42$, $p \leq .001$

and in age $F(4, 1483) = 13.77$, $p \leq .001$. Univariate analyses revealed significant differences between males and females in Self-Criticism, $F(1, 1486) = 18.44$, $p \leq .001$, Vulnerability, $F(1, 1486) = 38.68$, $p \leq .001$, and Perceived Lack of Competence $F(1, 1486) = 4.10$, $p \leq .05$, but not in Anxiety. Girls report higher levels of Self-Criticism,Vulnerability, and Perceived Lack of Competence than do boys (see Figure, 5).

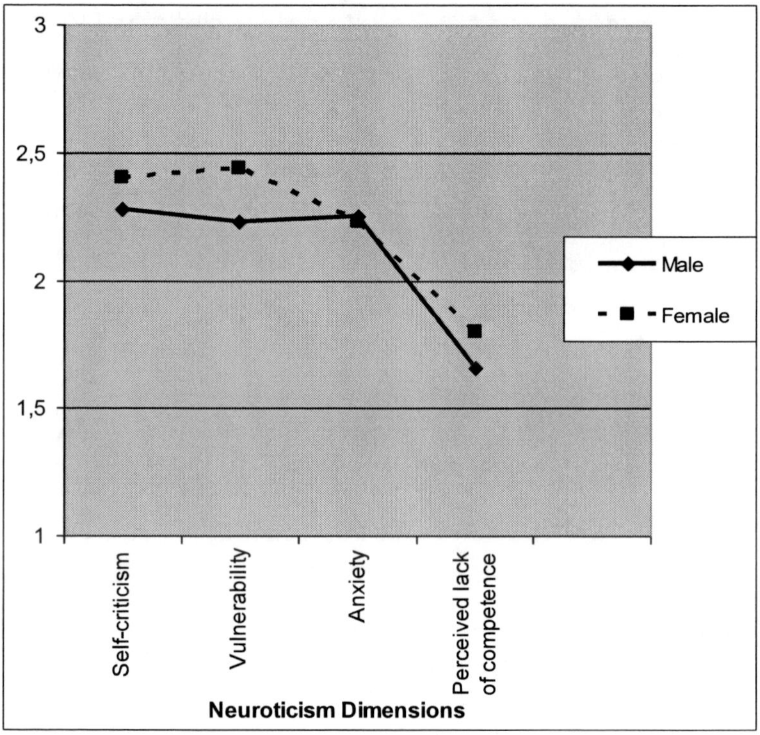

Figure 5. Comparison of neuroticism dimensions according to gender.

Univariate analyses revealed significant differences between children and adolescents in Self-Criticism, $F(1, 1486) = 13.90$, $p \leq .001$, Vulnerability, $F(1, 1486) = 4.35$, $p \leq .05$ and Anxiety $F(1, 1486) = 43.57$, $p \leq .001$, although no significant differences in Perceived Lack of Competence were reached. Children report higher levels of Self-Criticism,Vulnerability, and Anxiety than do adolescents (see Figure, 6).

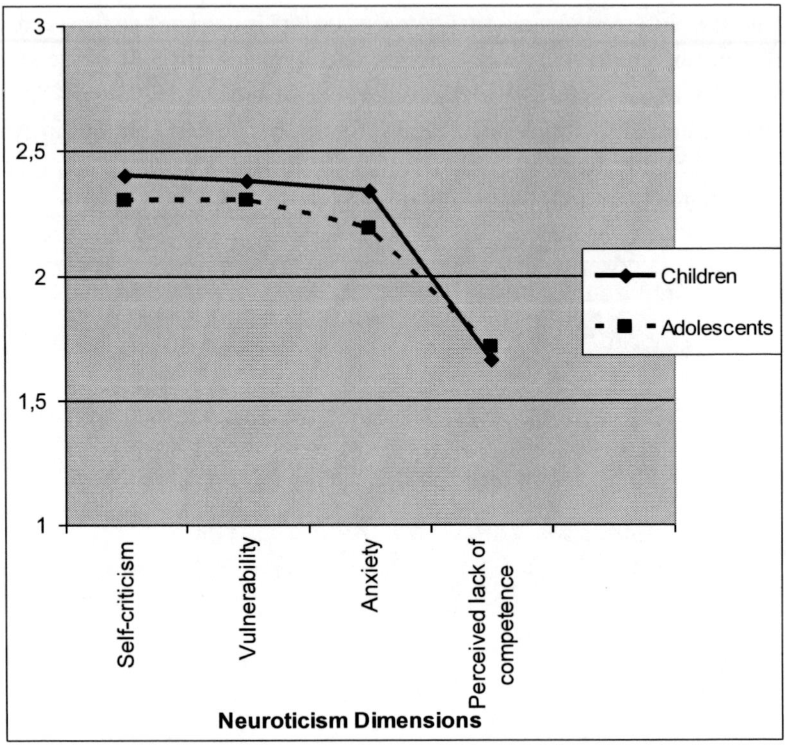

Figure 6. Comparison of neuroticism dimensions according to age.

The Relationship of Parenting Styles As Perceived by Children with Neuroticism According to Gender and Ages

Two multiple regression analyses were performed for each gender separately, to test the relations of parental styles (mothers' and fathers' acceptance, pathological control, and extreme autonomy) with neuroticism, while controlling for age.

The global prediction for neuroticism was significant for male, $F(6, 667) = 22.73$, $p \leq .001$ and for female $F(6, 791) = 9.80$, $p \leq .001$. The model explained 17 % of the variance of male neuroticism and 7% of variance of female neuroticism. In all cases (girls and boys) only mother and father pathological control was significant predictor of neuroticism (see Table 2).

Table 2. Summary of multiple regression analyses of parental styles on neuroticism in male and female (controlling for age)

Dependent	Predictors	Beta	t	P
Neuroticism (Male)	Acceptance Father	-.02	-.42	*n.s.*
	Pathological Control Father	.24	4.93	.001
	Extreme Autonomy Father	.02	.38	*n.s.*
	Acceptance Mother	.01	.21	*n.s.*
	Pathological Control Mother	.22	4.65	.001
	Extreme Autonomy Mother	-.06	-1.38	*n.s.*
Neuroticism (Female)	Acceptance Father	-.04	-1.1	*n.s.*
	Pathological Control Father	.11	2.46	.01
	Extreme Autonomy Father	.03	.78	*n.s.*
	Acceptance Mother	-.01	-.18	*n.s.*
	Pathological Control Mother	.17	3.84	.001
	Extreme Autonomy Mother	.01	-.05	*n.s.*

CONCLUSION

Several authors have underscored the importance of parenting for behaviour and personality development in children (Ivanova and Israel, 2006; Gaylord, Kitzmann, and Coleman, 2003; Richaud, Mesurado, and Lemos, 2012).

However, it is not the parental style reported by parents or observed externally that truly influences children, but rather that perceived and reported by children themselves (Schaefer, 1965; Richaud de Minzi, 2007; Samper, Cortés, Mestre, Nácher, and Tur, 2006). On the other hand, previous studies have shown that perceived parenting styles of both mothers and fathers change according to the gender and age of the children (Rodríguez, Del Barrio, and Carrasco, 2009).

In this sense, the first objective pursued by the current study was to identify the differences in parenting styles (in mothers and fathers) as perceived by boys and girls during childhood and adolescence. The results indicate that in effect, mother and father parenting styles are perceived in a different way by children and adolescents, according to their gender. Males perceive greater levels of extreme autonomy and pathological control, than females, from both fathers and mothers. These results coincide with those of other studies, which have shown that boys perceive their parents to be both stricter (Gaylord, Kitzmann, and Coleman, 2003; Sorbring, Rödholm-Funnemark, and Palmerus, 2003) and more negligent than their female sisters do (Hines, Kantor, and Holt, 2006), which would appear to respond to cultural influences on parenting. Parents would tend to give more freedom to boys than to girls, while at the same time punishing boys more severely if they fail to live up to a family norm or if they fail to reach the goals established in the family environment.

Mothers, fathers, and families in general interact with their children based on their cultural beliefs and values. Cultural differences in the definitions of sensitivity and responsiveness affect how parents rear and relate to their children (Reebye, Ross, and Jamieson, 1999). Cultural differences in the expectations of children at each stage of development might also lead to varying patterns of parent-child interactions and differential child outcomes (Richaud, 2010). The results of this study and of prior studies are written within Western cultural contexts with patterns that broadly coincide. It would be interesting to analyze whether these patterns vary among cultures, such as Oriental culture, for example. In the case of parental acceptance (both from mother and father) no differences were found between girls and boys, which leads to the assumption that sons and daughters perceive the same support, communication and affection from both parents.

In relation to the age of the children, it was observed that the children perceived higher levels of acceptance, pathological control and extreme autonomy than did adolescents, both from their father and their mother. However, it should be noted that the differences found between children and adolescents with respect to extreme autonomy (both in the father and the mother) and of acceptance from the mother, are less than in relation to pathological control.

The children perceived greater affection, involvement, communication and supervision both from fathers and mothers, as well as higher levels of control through punishments, strict supervision of their activities or retreat from relationships on their part.

Children seem to perceive that their parents exercises higher levels of pathological control over them than do adolescents because it is probable that adolescents rebel from this type of parental practices, to which parents would be obliged to adjust their parenting style.

The parent-child relationship doesn't diminish in importance after primary school, but rather takes on new characteristics. As children grow up, the opportunities for conflict and lack of comprehension increase, because parents are not always successful at adjusting their parenting practices to the development of autonomy among older children and adolescents (Marcoen and Brumagne, 1985). Parents, and adults on general, are seen as having less capacity for acceptance and as being more likely to act as experts or in an authoritarian style which impedes the reflexion process that young people prefer in order to discuss their emotional problems and their fears with friends and peers (Richaud, Moreno, and Sacchi, 2011).

The second goal of this research was to analyse the differences in neuroticism dimensions (self-criticism, vulnerability, anxiety, perceived lack of competence), according to gender and age. The current study has shown that females report higher levels of neuroticism, especially self-criticism, vulnerability and perceived lack of competence. These results line up with research undertaken with adult populations that showed that females scored higher on neuroticism than men, even in different cultures (Chapman, Duberstein, Sörensen, and Lyness, 2007; Weisberg, DeYoung, and Hirsh, 2011). They also found that these differences were maintained across different points in the lifespan which is consistent with the notion that biological and sociocultural forces responsible for this gender differentiation are present since childhood and do not diminish in old age (Chapman, Duberstein, Sörensen, and Lyness, 2007). It is worth mentioning that differences were not found in male's and female's anxiety levels, which differs from the findings of other studies, which consistently find that females report higher levels of anxiety than males do (Lowe and Reynolds, 2006; Soto, John, Gosling, and Potter, 2011). Furthermore, the results shown that children who show demonstrate higher levels of self-criticism, vulnerability and anxiety than adolescents. This could be due to maturational changes which allow adolescents to acquire higher levels of emotional stability along with resulting reductions in vulnerability and anxiety (Srivastava, John, Gosling, and Potter, 2003; Soto, John, Gosling, and Potter, 2011).

The third objective of this chapter was to study the relationship between perceived parenting styles with children neuroticism according to gender and ages.

Several studies have found that ill-adapted family environments partly explain dysfunctional in children (Loeber and Hay, 1997). In our study, we found that the only parenting dimension that is associated with neuroticism is pathological control, that is, excessive, intrusive control, based on guilt, which implies the implementation of strict norms, punishments and scolding, based on a negative evaluation of the child and distancing through rejection. These results are to be expected given that the use of excessively strict and coercive discipline directed at controlling children and making them submissive, all of which paralyzes them emotionally (Richaud de Minzi, 2006b). Such parents are demanding, strict, give punishments and do not allow children to express their opinions. They do not like authority to be questioned, they establish very high standards and demand that these standards be met. These parents value submissiveness and obedience and discourage independence and individuality. In this way, they can bring about lack of self-confidence, hypercontrol and low self-esteem in children, which causes them difficulty in making decisions for themselves, even when acting in a socially acceptable way (Allès-Jardel, Fourdrinier, Roux, and Schneider, 2002; Richaud, Mesurado, Samper, Llorca, Lemos, and Tur, 2013).

It is of interest that parental acceptance didn't appear negatively related to neuroticism, that is, actually as a defence against emotional instability, given that there is evidence that parental acceptance, manifested through warm relationships and positive interactions with children and inversely with emotional instability and neuroticism (Richaud et al., in press).

On the other hand, it was to be expected that extreme autonomy would not be strongly related to neuroticism, given that complete autonomy with insufficient parental supervision of children's activities has been associated mainly with antisocial and deviant behaviour (Dishion, 1990; Allès-Jardel, Fourdrinier, Roux, and Schneider, 2002) more than hypercontrol and emotional instability as a difficulty to give an adequate answer to the magnitude of the stimulus.

REFERENCES

Allès-Jardel, M., Fourdrinier, C., Roux, A., and Schneider, B. H. (2002). Parents' structuring of children's daily lives in relation to the quality and stability of children's friendships. *International Journal of Psychology,* 37, 65–73.

Baumrind, D. (1991). The influence of parenting style on adolescent competence and substance use. *Journal of Early Adolescence,* 11(1), 56-95.

Belsky, J. (1990). Parental and nonparental child care and children's socio-emotional development: A decade in review. *Journal of Marriage and the Family*, 52, 885-903.

Belsky, J., Jaffee, S. R., Caspi, A., Moffitt, T., and Silva, P. A. (2003). International relationships in young adulthood and their life course, mental health, and personality correlates. *Journal of Family Psychology,* 17, 460–471.

Blehar, M. C. and Oren, D. A. (1999). *Gender Differences in Depression. Medscape-Mental Health,* 1(2). Available at: http://www.medscape.com/viewpublication/125_toc?vol=1andiss=2. Accessed: October 2nd, 2008.

Bruck, C. S. and Allen, T. D. (2003) The relationship between big five personality traits, negative affectivity, type A behavior, and work–family conflict. *Journal of Vocational Behavior,* 63, 457–472.

Bugental, D. B. and Grusec, J. E. (2006) Socialization processes. In: N. Eisenberg, W. Damon and R. L. Lerner (Eds.). *Handbook of child psychology. Social, emotional, and personality development* (Vol. 3, pp. 366–428). New York: Wiley.

Burbach, D. J. and Borduin, C. M. (1986). Parent-child relations and the etiology of depression: A review of methods and findings. *Clinical Psychology Review*, 6, 133-153.

Canli T., Zhao Z., Desmond, J. E., Kang, E., Gross, J., and Gabrieli, J. D. (2001) An fMRI study of personality influences on brain reactivity to emotional stimuli. *Behavioral Neuroscience,* 115(1), 33–42.

Costa Jr., P. T. and McCrae, R. R. (1980) Influence of extraversion and neuroticism on subjective well-being: Happy and unhappy people. *Journal of Personality and Social Psychology,* 38(4), 668–678.

Costa Jr., P. T. and McCrae, R. R. (1991). *NEO PI-R. Professional manual. Revised NEO personality inventory (NEO PI-R) and NEO five-factor inventory (NEO-FFI)*. US: Psychological Assesment Resources, Inc.

Costa Jr., P. T. and McCrae, R. R. (2006). Age changes in personality and their origins: Comment on Roberts, Walton, and Viechtbauer (2006). *Psychological Bulletin,* 1(132), 26–28.

Chapman, B. P., Duberstein, P. R., Sörensen, S., and Lyness, J. M. (2007). Gender differences in five factor model personality traits in an elderly cohort: Extension of robust and surprising findings to an older generation. *Personality and Individual Differences* 43(6), 1594–1603.

Chico Librán, E. (2006). Personality dimensions and subjective well-being. *The Spanish Journal of Psychology,* 9(1), 38–44.

Craske, M. G. (1999) *Anxiety disorders: Psychological approaches to theory and treatment.* Boulder, CO: Westview Press.

Darling, N. and Steinberg, L. (1993). Parenting style as context: An integrative model. *Psychological Bulletin,* 113(3), 487- 496.

Dishion, T. J. (1990). The ecology of boys' peer relations in middle school. *Child Development,* 61, 874–892.

Eysenck, H. J. (1967) *The biological basis of personality*. Springfield, IL: Thomas.

Gaylord, N. K., Kitzmann, M. and Coleman, J. K. (2003). Parent and children's perceptions of parental behaviour: associations with children's psychological adjustment in the classroom. *Parenting: Science and Practice,* 3(1), 23-47.

Goldberg, D. (2001) Vulnerability factors for common mental illnesses. *The British Journal of Psychiatry,* 40, 69–71.

Hansenne, M., Reggers, J., Pinto, E., Kjiri, K., Ajamier, A., and Ansseau, M. (1999) Temperament and character inventory (TCI) and depression. *Journal of Psychiatric Research,* 33(1), 31–36.

Hines, D., Kantor, G. and Holt, M. (2006) Similarities in siblings' experiences of neglectful parenting behaviours. *Child Abuse and Neglect,* 30, 619-637.

Ivanova, M. and Israel, A. (2006). Family stability as a protective factor against psychopathology for urban children receiving psychological services. *Journal of Clinical Child and Adolescent Psychology,* 35, 564–570.

Johnson, B. M., Shulman, S. and Collins, W. A. (1991). Systemic patterns of parenting as reported by adolescents: developmental differences and implications for psychosocial outcomes. *Journal of Adolescent Research,* 16, 235–252.

Judge, T. A. and Ilies, R. (2002). Relationship of personality to performance motivation: A meta-analytic review. *Journal of Applied Psychology,* 87, 797–807.

Judge T. A., Locke E. A. and Durham C. C. (1997). The dispositional causes of job satisfaction: A core evaluations approach. *Research in Organizational Behavior,* 19, 151–188.

Krueger, R. F., Caspi, A. and Moffitt, T. E. (2000) Epidemiological personology: The unifying role of personality in population-based research on problem behaviors. *Journal of Personality,* 68(6), 967–98.

Lahey, B. B. (2009). Public health significance of neuroticism. *American Psychologist,* 64, 241–256.

Larsen, R. J. and Ketelaar, T. (1989) Extraversion, neuroticism, and susceptibility to positive and negative mood induction procedures. *Personality and Individual Differences,* 10(12), 1221–1228.

Larsen, R. J. and Ketelaar, T. (1991) Personality and susceptibility to positive and negative emotional states. *Journal of Personality and Social Psychology,* 61(1), 132–140.

Lemos, V. (2006). La evaluación de la personalidad infantil a partir del enfoque de los cinco grandes factores de personalidad (Big Five). *Psicodiagnosticar,* 16, 97–108.

Loeber, R. and Hay, D. (1997) Key issues in the development of aggression and violence from childhood to early adulthood. *Annual Review of Psychology,* 48, 371-410.

Lowe, P. A. and Reynolds, C. R. (2006). Examination of the psychometric properties of the Adult Manifest Anxiety Scale-Elderly Version (AMAS-E) scores. *Educational and Psychological Measurement,* 66, 93-115.

Maccoby, E. E. and Martin, J. (1983). Socialization in the content of the family. In: P. H. Mussen and E. M. Hetherington (Eds.), *Handbook of Child Psychology Socialization, Personality, and Social Development* (4th ed., Vol. 4.). New York: John Wiley.

Marcoen, A. and Brumagne, M. (1985). Loneliness among children and young adolescents. *Developmental Psychology*, 21, 1025-1031.

McCrae, R. R., Costa, P. T., Terracciano, A., Parker, W. D., Mills, C. J., De Fruyt, F., and Mervielde, I. (2002) Personality trait development from age 12 to age 18: Longitudinal, cross-sectional, and cross-cultural analyses. *Journal of Personality and Social Psychology,* 83(6), 1456–1468.

McCrae, R., R., Costa Jr., P. T., Hrebícková, M., Urbánek, T., Martin, T., Oryol, V., Rukavishnikov, A. A., and Senin, I. G. (2004). Age differences in personality traits across cultures: Self-report and observer perspectives. *European Journal of Personality,* 18, 143-157.

Mesurado, B. and Richaud de Minzi, M. C. (2013). Child's personality and perception of parental relationship as correlates of optimal experience. *Journal of Happiness Studies,* 14(1), 199-214.

Mesurado, B. and Richaud, M. C. (In press). Children's perception of parental relationship and personality traits in Argentinean children. In: E. E. Crossman and M. A. Weiler (Eds.), *Personality Traits: Causes, Conceptions and Consequences*. New York: Nova Science Publishers.

Mestre, M. V., Samper, P., Tur, A. M., and Díez, I. (2001). Estilos de Crianza y Desarrollo de Prosocialidad en los Hijos. *Revista de Psicología General y Aplicada,* 54(4), 691-703.

Naquin, S. S. and Holton, E. F. I. (2002). The effects of personality, affectivity, and work commitment on motivation to improve work through learning. *Human Resource Development Quarterly,* 13, 357–376.

Norman, J. E. and Streiner, D. L. (1994). *Biostatistics. The Bare Essentials*. St Louis, Missoury: Mosby.

Reebye, P. N., Ross, S. E. and Jamieson, K. (1999). A review of the literature on the development of attachment theory and the study of cross-cultural practices influencing attachment [Online].Accessed: http://www.attachmentacrosscultures.org/research/.

Reynaud, E., El Khoury-Malhame, M., Rossier, J., Blin, O., and Khalfa, S. (2012). Neuroticism modifies psychophysiological responses to fearful films. *PLoS ONE,* 7(3), e32413. doi:10.1371/journal.pone.0032413.

Richaud, M. C., Lemos, V. and Mesurado, B. (2011). Relaciones entre la percepción que tienen los niños de los estilos de relación y de la empatía de los padres y la conducta prosocial en la niñez media y tardía. *Avances en Psicología. Latinoamericana,* 29(2), 330-343.

Richaud, M. C., Mesurado, B. and Lemos, V. (2012). Links between perception of parental actions and prosocial behavior in early adolescence. *Journal of Child and Family Studies*. DOI: 10.1007/s10826-012-9617-x

Richaud, M. C., Moreno, J. E. and Sacchi, C. (2011). Un modelo acerca de la relación entre los vínculos interpersonales y el afrontamiento en la adolescencia. In: M. C. Richaud and V. Lemos (Eds.), *Psicología y otras Ciencias del Comportamiento. Compendio de investigaciones actuales* (Vol. 1, pp. 137-157). Ediciones CIIPME-CONICET y Universidad Adventista del Plata Ediciones.

Richaud, M. C., Mesurado, B., Samper-García, P., Llorca, A., and Tur, A. (2003). Estilos parentales, inestabilidad emocional y agresividad en niños de nivel socioeconómico bajo en Argentina y España. *Ansiedad y Estrés,* 19(1), 43-69.

Richaud de Minzi, M. C. (2006a). Stress and coping in adolescence. In: A. M. Columbus (Ed.), *Advances in Psychology Research* (Vol. 45, pp. 67-84). Hauppauge, NY: Nova Editorial Publishers, Inc.

Richaud de Minzi, M. C. (2006b). Loneliness and depression in middle and late childhood: Its relationship to attachment and parental styles. *Journal of Genetic Psychology,* 167(2), 189-210.

Richaud de Minzi, M. C. (2007). La percepción de estilos de relación con su padre y madre en niños y niñas de 8 a 12 años. *Revista Iberoamericana de Diagnóstico y Evaluación Psicológica,* 1(23), 63-81.

Roberts, B. W., Walton, K. E. and Viechtbauer, W. (2005). Patterns of mean-level change in personality traits across the life course: a meta-analysis of longitudinal studies. *Psychological Bulletin,* 132(1), 1-25.

Robinson, M. D., Ode, S., Moeller, S. K., and Goetz, P. W. (2007) Neuroticism and affective priming: evidence for a neuroticism-linked negative schema. *Personality and individual differences,* 42(7), 1221–1231.

Rodríguez, M. A., Del Barrio, M. V. and Carrasco, M. A. (2009). ¿Cómo perciben los hijos la crianza materna y paterna? Diferencias por edad y sexo. *Escritos de Psicología,* 2(2), 10-18.

Rothbaum, F. and Weisz, J. (1994). Parental converging and child externalizing behavior in nonclinical samples: A meta-analysis. *Psychological Bulletin,* 116, 55–74.

Ruble, D. N., Greulich, F., Pomerantz, E. M., and Gochberg, B. (1993). The role of gender-related processes in the development of sex differences in self-evaluation and depression. *Journal of Affective Disorders,* 29, 97-128.

Samper, P., Cortés, M. T., Mestre, V., Nácher, M. J., and Tur, A. M. (2006). Adaptación del Child´s Report of Parent Behavior Inventory a población Española. *Psicothema* 18(2), 263-271.

Schaefer, E. S. (1965). Children's reports of parental behavior: an inventory. *Child Development,* 36(2), 413-424.

Schneewind, K. A. and Kupsch, M. (2007). Patterns of neuroticism, work-family stress, and resources as determinants of personal distress: A cluster analysis of young, dual-earner families at the individual and couple level. *Journal of Individual Differences,* 28, 150–160.

Shaffer, D. R. (2009). *Social and Personality Development.* Belmond, CA: Wadsworth.

Skinner, E., Johnson, S. and Snyder, T. (2005). Six dimensions of parenting: A motivational model. *Parenting: Science and Practice,* 2, 175–235.

Soto, C. J., John, O. P., Gosling, S. D., and Potter, J. (2011). Age differences in personality traits from 10 to 65: Big five domains and facets in a large cross-sectional sample. *Journal of Personality and Social Psychology,* 100 (2), 330–348.

Sorbring, E., Rödholm-Funnemark, M. and Palmerus, K. (2003) Boys´and gilrs´ perceptions of parental discipline in transgression situations. *Infant and Child Development,* 12, 53-69.

Spinath, F. M. and O'Connor, T. G. (2003). A behavioral genetic study of the overlap between personality and parenting. *Journal of Personality,* 71(5), 785-808.

Srivastava, S., John, O. P., Gosling, S. D., and Potter, J. (2003). Development of personality in early and middle adulthood: Set like plaster or persistent change? *Journal of Personality and Social Psychology,* 84, 1041–1053.

Stewart, M. E., Ebmeier, K. P. and Deary, I. J. (2005) Personality correlates of happiness and sadness: EPQ-R and TPQ compared. *Personality and individual differences*. 38, 1085–1096.

Swickert, R. and Owens, T. (2010). The interaction between neuroticism and gender influences the perceived availability of social support. *Personality and Individual Differences,* 48(4), 385-390.

Van Os, J. and Jones, P. B. (1999) Early risk factors and adult person-environment relationships in affective disorder. *Psychological Medicine,* 29(5), 1055–1067.

Weisberg, Y. J., DeYoung, C. G. and Hirsh, J. B. (2011). Gender differences in personality across the ten aspects of the Big Five. *Frontiers in Psychology,* 2(178), 1-11.

Wolfradt, U., Hempel, S. and Miles, J. N. V. (2003). Perceived parenting style, depersonalisation, anxiety and coping behaviour in adolescents. *Personality and Individual Differences,* 34, 521-532.

In: Psychology of Neuroticism
Editor: Kristel Parn

ISBN: 978-1-62808-150-3

Chapter 3

NEUROTICISM AND RESILIENCE: EVALUATING MINDFULNESS AS A MEDIATOR

Keri Johns, David J. Chavers and Elise Labbé*
University of South Alabama, AL, US

ABSTRACT

Neuroticism is implicated in negative affect predictions, and functions as a complex dimension of personality, a vulnerability factor for psychopathology, and as the primary underlying factor in trait negative affect. The research literature's consensual acceptance of neuroticism as a factor in psychological distress is well documented through research studies and meta-analyses. Neuroticism is linked to deficiencies in emotional and cognitive functioning, resulting in problems with self-regulation, attention and awareness. Neuroticism has demonstrated inverse correlations with resilience: the perceived ability to cope effectively with adverse situations (Labbé et al., 2011, 2012). Ongoing research continues to explore psychosocial variables that can effectively mitigate neuroticism's negative effects. Mindfulness, as a psychological construct and intervention based on a core spiritual practice of Buddhism, has gained acceptance in recent years due to its positive

* Correspondence concerning this article should be addressed to Elise E. Labbé, Ph.D. Department of Psychology, University of South Alabama, Mobile, AL 36688 elabbe@usouthal.edu.

effects on a variety of psychological stressors (Baer, 2006), and its potential as an effective mediator of neuroticism (Feltman et al., 2009; Fetterman et al., 2010; Labbé et al., 2011, 2012). The cognitive qualities and emotional outcomes of mindfulness may produce mediation effects on the ineffective attention and awareness that leads to negative reactivity in neuroticism, and provide a stronger relationship with subjective resilience. Findings of recent research regarding neuroticism, mindfulness, and resilience are presented in a discussion of a mindfulness model to mitigate the effects of neuroticism on resilience. Future directions of research and strengths and limitations of current research are discussed.

INTRODUCTION

A conceptualization of mindfulness as a mediator of neuroticism leading to increased resilience can begin with a stress and response cycle. It is the individual's response to the experience of stressors that produces either psychological well-being or distress, either of which, have reinforcing properties that often perpetuate an ongoing adaptive cycle of stress and response. Neuroticism occurs within an individual's psychological reality regardless of other stressors, and higher levels of neuroticism are known to produce negative affect judgments about stressors. The neurotic affect experience of stress, compounds the internal distress of experience, and can alter the behavioral response to the stressor. An individual's response to a particular internal experience can be viewed as an adaptive coping mechanism, and successful adaptation can be viewed as increasing the individual's resilience, or as reducing the distress in order to facilitate healthy functioning. In this conceptualization of stress and response, adaptive factors, which may facilitate increased individual resilience, are of prime interest for both the researcher and the clinician.

Mindfulness, as a psychological construct of present focused attention and awareness in a particular way, has gained acceptance in recent years due to its positive effects on a variety of psychological stressors (Baer, 2006). Those positive effects includes its potential as an effective mediator of neuroticism (Feltman, Robinson, and Ode, 2009; Fetterman, Robinson, Ode, and Gordon, 2010; Labbé, Womble, and Shenesey, 2011; Labbé, Womble, Shenesey, Chavers, and Wilson, 2012). The cognitive qualities and emotional outcomes of mindfulness may produce mediation effects on the ineffective attention and awareness that leads to negative reactivity in neuroticism, and provide a stronger relationship with resilience. In this chapter, we present findings of recent research regarding neuroticism, mindfulness, and resilience. We will also discuss mediation or moderator models of mindfulness in relation to neuroticism and resilience.

METHOD

The published research literature was found using PsychInfo, Pubmed, and Google Scholar, as well as looking through the reference sections of relevant articles. Search keywords used to find articles were "mindfulness", "resilience", "neurotic", "self-regulation", "emotion regulation", "psychological "distress", "trauma", and "coping" and combinations of these terms. There was no date restrictions prior to 2013 placed on the searches, such that all potentially related articles were located, regardless of research date. Only research written in English was used and studies were included that used small samples and quasi-experimental designs. Finally, only studies that specifically used, measured, or evaluated "mindfulness" or "resilience" were considered for inclusion. Other types of meditation and relaxation practices were not included. Four meta-analyses and 29 studies meeting these criteria were included in the current review.

NEUROTICISM AND PSYCHOLOGICAL DISTRESS

Neuroticism is a well-established construct implicated in a range of negative emotional health predictions and functions as a complex dimension of personality, a vulnerability factor for psychopathology, and as the primary underlying factor in trait negative affect. Neuroticism as a personality trait is fundamental to understanding and predicting human behavior (Fetterman et al., 2010). Costa and McCrae (1980) describe neuroticism as one of the broadest and most pervasive domains of personality and as being a factor in maladaptive psychological functioning. In the NEO model of personality consisting of Neuroticism, Extroversion and Openness (Costa and McCrae, 1992), neuroticism represents a stable contrast to adjustment or emotional stability, and describes the tendency of individuals to experience negative affect across time or situations. The underlying facets of neuroticism are anxiety, angry hostility, depression, self-consciousness, impulsiveness of control, and vulnerability to stress with each facet implicated in research regarding negative affect and lower life satisfaction (Costa, McCrae, and Holland, 1984).

Research in recent years continues to provide support for the effect of neuroticism on psychological distress. Studies by Barnhofer, Duggan, and Griffith (2011), and Feltman et al., (2009) provide support for the relationship of neuroticism with anxiety and depression. Fetterman et al. (2010) reported that impulsiveness of control, along with angry hostility and self-consciousness, are aspects of behavioral dysregulation that were associated with neuroticism. Lent and Schwartz (2012) reported that professional counselors with higher levels of neuroticism were more vulnerable to stress, and therefore emotional exhaustion, than counselors who had lower levels of neuroticism. These recent studies, as well as others, indicate neuroticism's continued and well established link to psychological distress, and point to the importance of the individual levels of the underlying facets involved in neuroticism. These facets are instrumental in the experience of negative affect and can be expressed as emotional instability or maladjustment, or as a lack of effective self-regulation.

NEUROTICISM AND RESILIENCE

The opposite of high neuroticism is lower anxiety, less pervasive anger and frustration, greater mood stability, lower shame and embarrassment, greater control over cravings and urges, and more confidence in coping with stress (Costa and McCrae, 1992). The description of these contrasting emotional and cognitive reactions to high neuroticism implies a well-adjusted and emotionally stable individual, or a description of a person who is highly resilient despite adversity. Resilience is the ability to cope effectively with adversity across time and allows individuals to recover faster and demonstrate better social and emotional coping in stressful situations (Labbé, et al., 2011).

Positive coping, or resilience, implies an adaptive response to difficulty. Pargament (1997) describes coping as an attempt to preserve that, which is of significance, in stressful circumstances. Pargament and Brant (1998) also describe the attempt to preserve a significant value as maximizing it when dealing with stressors. Significant values, according to Pargament and Brant, depend upon the individual's concept of value, and can be positive or negative, psychological, social, physical, material, or spiritual. Research indicates unique factors that influence a person's response to stressors or traumatic events, meaning that individuals respond differently to stressors or traumatic events (Labbé et al., 2012). Factors that could inhibit resilience or adaptive coping include low socioeconomic status (SES), life stress, low intelligence, minority race status, childhood abuse, and the lack of education, or social support, and past trauma and/or psychiatric problems. Factors that could work to enhance resilience or adaptive coping include the inverse of the qualities of risk factors (e.g., higher SES, social support, lack of psychiatric history, higher education, and race) (Brewin, Andrews, and Valentine, 2000). Enhancement factors of resilience could also include self-efficacy, a positive outlook, courage, cognitive flexibility, humor, social skills, spirituality, and others as well (Bonanno, 2004; Neenan, 2009). The impact of risk and protective factors on resilience indicates that resilience is not only a contrast to emotional instability, maladjustment, or a lack of effective self-regulation but is its own construct to be studied and enhanced (Friborg, Barlaug, Martinussen, Rosenvinge, and Hjemdal, 2005).

Research on psychological constructs or theories that assume individual differences based on experience or the influence of factors in response to stressors or more mundane life situations, often is strengthened by the consideration of personality factors. Adaptation-Level (AL) theory (see Costa and McCrae, 1980), posited a similar stance regarding successful adjustment in situations that effected subjective well-being or happiness. AL theory states that the individual's past experience accounted for much of the person's efficacy at effectively adjusting to current situations. Costa and McCrae (1980) found that while individual experience did account for a large portion of the variance in adjustment for happiness, the personality traits of neuroticism and extroversion were necessary as well to complete the model. McCrae (1999) adhered to this theoretical position when he posited that religion and spirituality, individual difference constructs dependent upon experience or influential factors, should be studied in the light of the individual personality differences. In the model of individual differences, individual levels of resilience can be studied in the light of individual personality levels. The various factors that influence subjective resilience may be influenced by the individual's level of neuroticism in the experience of stressors, affecting the implementation of adaptive coping responses.

Research regarding resilience supports the influence of personality domains on individual levels of self-perceived resilience across various resilience measures, with neuroticism demonstrating the strongest relationship with resilience—a consistently negative association (Labbé et al., 2012). One of the oldest resilience measures, the Resilience Scale (RS; Wagnild and

Young, 1993), demonstrated resilience to be negatively associated with depression and positively associated with self-actualization and stress management, constructs that embody the underlying facets of neuroticism. A cross validation study on the Resilience Scale for Adults (RSA; Hjemdal, Friborg, Martinussen, and Rosenvinge, 2001) revealed a strong positive association with emotional stability as the inverse of neuroticism (Friborg et al., 2005). Two recent studies using the Resilience Questionnaire (RQ; Sideroff, 2004) also found strong negative associations between resilience and neuroticism (Labbé et al., 2011; 2012). Research supports the idea that neuroticism is a risk factor for psychological well-being, and has a negative association with the independent construct of resilience, a form of effective coping in the face of adversity. Existing research does not provide much insight into the particular mechanisms that are involved in the consistent relationship between personality and resilience, or if and how those constructs can influence each other. Research evaluating these mechanisms or mediators or moderations of resilience in relation to neuroticism would further our understanding of why some individuals are more resilient than others. Furthermore, understanding these processes may facilitate the development of interventions for increasing resilience even when an individual may experience greater levels of neuroticism.

Mindfulness, Neuroticism, and Resilience

Mechanisms explaining the established relationship between neuroticism and resilience need to be explored further. One such construct that may explain this relationship is mindfulness. Being mindful can be described as having a present-focused awareness. A mindful person is one that is attentive of the present moment in an accepting and nonjudging way (Kabat-Zinn, 1990). Part of being mindful is the ability to be aware one's current thoughts, feelings, sensations, and other inner experiences without judging them as good or bad and not immediately reacting to these experiences. Mindfulness is proposed to account for the relationship between neuroticism and resilience because of its recent research support for its relationships to both of these constructs. As a trait, mindfulness is associated with positive psychological outcomes and it is inversely associated with psychological distress. Specifically, previous research literature on mindfulness supports its inverse relationship with anger, depression, and anxiety and a positive relationship with psychological constructs such as optimism, self-esteem, and self-compassion (Dekeyser, Raes, Leijssen, Leysen, and Dewulf, 2008; Keng, Smoski, and Robins, 2011; Brown and Ryan, 2003). Additionally, trait mindfulness has been shown to relate to positive interpersonal outcomes such as less social anxiety, decreased affliction from others' distress (Dekeyser et al., 2008), increased empathy, increased emotion regulation abilities (Block-Lerner, Adair, Plumb, Rhatigan, and Orsillo, 2007; Dekeyser et al., 2008; Wachs and Cordova, 2007). Mindfulness-based interventions have been shown to foster trait mindfulness as well as these positive psychological outcomes (Carmody and Baer, 2008; Hofmann, Sawyer, Witt, and Oh, 2010; Keng et al., 2011). Furthermore, the level of trait mindfulness is positively associated with the amount of meditation experience and practice (Baer, Lykins, and Peters, 2012; Carmody and Baer, 2008; Keng et al., 2011), suggesting that mindfulness as a trait is indeed malleable. Additional evidence of this comes from meta-analyses examining the effectiveness of mindfulness-based therapies (Hofmann et al., 2010; Keng et al, 2011). Randomized controlled trials of mindfulness-based interventions, including Mindfulness-Based Stress Reduction (MBSR), Mindfulness-Based Cognitive Therapy (MBCT), Dialectical Behavior Therapy (DBT), and Acceptance and Commitment Therapy (ACT), have reported success at increasing mindfulness and positive mental health outcomes (Keng et al., 2011, Labbé, 2011), as well as progress in treatment for several psychological disorders including anxiety and depression (Hofmann et al., 2010; Keng et al, 2011).

Given the positive outcomes associated with mindfulness, it would be expected that mindfulness would be positively related to resilience and inversely related to neuroticism. Similarly, mindfulness may provide intervention opportunities for people high in neuroticism and prevention opportunities promoting future resilience. Let us first examine the relationship between mindfulness and neuroticism.

Mindfulness and neuroticism. Given the relationship between trait mindfulness and mindfulness-based interventions decreasing psychological distress and emotion dysregulation, it is reasonable to expect that mindfulness would be inversely related to neuroticism. The current literature supports this relationship, suggesting that increased mindfulness is related to decreased neuroticism. A compelling meta-analysis examined available research studies of mindfulness and its relationship to different personality traits (Giluk, 2009). Trait mindfulness was most strongly related to neuroticism (inversely) out of the big five personality factors. It was also moderately inversely related to negative affect and positively associated with positive affect (Giluk, 2009). One possible limitation of this meta-analysis is the included studies did not all use the same mindfulness measures. This could be an issue as different measures examine different aspects of mindfulness. For example, the Mindfulness Attention Awareness Scale (MAAS; Brown and Ryan, 2003) focuses more on the attention and awareness aspects of being mindful, whereas the Five Facet Mindfulness Questionnaire encompasses the attentive and awareness aspects, but also includes other aspects of mindfulness such as nonreactivity and nonjudgment of the inner experience (FFMQ; Baer, Smith, Hopkins, Krietemeyer, and Toney, 2006b). Giluk (2009) addresses this as something that needs to be considered when measuring the construct of mindfulness. The acceptance and nonjudgment facets may be particularly salient in accounting for the relationship between mindfulness and neuroticism because they counter a neurotic interpretation of an event or experience (Giluk, 2009).

Additional support for a relationship between mindfulness and neuroticism is provided by several studies which evaluate the role of mindfulness in psychosocial models of neuroticism. One such study examining the relationship between neuroticism and behavior dysregulation, found that mindfulness mediated this relationship (Fetterman et al., 2010). That is, neuroticism was inversely related to mindfulness, which in turn was associated negatively with impulsivity and positively with self-control. Mindfulness was assessed with the MAAS (Brown and Ryan, 2003) in this study, suggesting that the lack of attention and awareness is the important element accounting for an individual being neurotic and impulsive or unable to regulate their behavior. When mindfulness is examined as a moderator of neuroticism with depressive symptoms, being high in mindfulness served as a protective factor for those high in neuroticism (Barnhofer et al., 2011; Feltman et al., 2009). Feltman et al. (2009) measured mindfulness utilizing the MAAS (Brown and Ryan, 2003), whereas Barnhofer et al. (2011) used the FFMQ (Baer et al., 2006). Thus, the awareness and attentional aspect of mindfulness proves to be important in both explorations, but support is provided for other valuable facets of being mindful, especially the ability to describe and label one's inner experience; having a nonjudgmental acceptance and nonreactivity to one's inner experience also appears to be relevant (Barnhofer et al., 2011). Additionally, increased mindfulness reduces the association between neuroticism and trait anger; those high in neuroticism that are also high in mindfulness have much lower trait anger (Feltman et al., 2009). Hence, a mindfulness-based intervention may be appropriate for people who score higher in neuroticism to help buffer from unhealthy psychological outcomes. Further support for the utility of mindfulness-based interventions is provided by a comparison between mindfulness meditation practitioners and matched controls (van den Hurk, Wingens, Giomi, Barendregt, Speckens, and van Schie, 2011).

Consistent with previously mentioned studies (e.g., Baer et al., 2012), trait mindfulness is increased as mindfulness-based practices such as meditation are increased (van den Hurk et al., 2011). While the difference between groups on neuroticism was not significantly different, increased meditation practice was significantly related to decreased neuroticism in those that practiced mindfulness meditation. Moreover, this relationship between more mindfulness meditation experience and lessened neuroticism is mediated by the mindfulness skills of awareness and nonjudging acceptance of one's experience (van den Hurk et al., 2011). Likewise, people having attended an intensive mindfulness retreat compared to a matched waitlist control group demonstrated an increase in mindfulness, perceived control, telomerase activity, and a decrease in neuroticism (Jacobs, Epel, Lin, Blackburn, Wolkowitz, Bridwell, Zanesco, Aichele, Sahdra, MacLean, King, Shaver, Rosenberg, Ferrer, Wallace, and Saron, 2011). Not only did increased mindfulness meditation practice decrease neuroticism, this relationship was accounted for by increased trait mindfulness, corroborating this discussion on a proposed mindfulness intervention for those higher in neuroticism. Trait mindfulness also accounted for the increase in perceived control, an important construct in resilience. The effect of meditation on increased telomerase activity was accounted for by decreased neuroticism, increased perceived control, and increased purpose in life. Decreased immune cell telomerase activity is a physical result from psychological stress and is associated with increased health risks (Jacobs et al., 2011). These studies support that mindfulness-based interventions show promise in decreasing neuroticism, as well as increasing resilience by increasing positive psychological outcomes, such as perceived control and purpose in life. Similarly, physical health resilience may be benefited as well, as exemplified by increased telomerase activity (Jacobs et al., 2011). This leads us into a discussion about the current literature associating mindfulness to resilience.

Mindfulness and resilience. In addition to the previously discussed inverse relationship between mindfulness and neuroticism, mindfulness is related positively to resilience and constructs associated with resilience. The current research literature overwhelmingly supports this link and it has been examined in different populations of people exposed to trauma. Mindful attention and awareness is associated with fewer post-traumatic stress disorder (PTSD) symptoms in adults exposed to trauma even when controlling for amount of traumatic events one is exposed to (Bernstein, Tanay, and Vujanovic, 2011). One study, which looked at professional American firefighters and PTSD symptoms, found similar results. Being mindfully attentive and aware was associated with not only fewer PTSD symptoms, but also fewer depressive symptoms, alcohol problems, and physical symptoms (Smith, et al., 2011). While most of these studies are correlational and therefore the directionality of effects cannot be determined, one study has explored being mindful as a preventative factor for Australian police officers (Williams, Ciarrochi, and Deane, 2010). The police officers were initially assessed while in their trainee phase and then again almost a year following graduation when they were working as officers (Williams et al., 2010). Trainees initially high in the attention and awareness aspects of mindfulness were less depressed a year later, even when controlling for their initial depression levels. Although this measure of mindfulness did not predict general mental health at follow-up, initial emotion identification did (Williams et al., 2010), which suggests that a different aspect of mindfulness such as the ability to describe one's thoughts, feelings, and emotions may be appropriate to include in future studies and that mindfulness as a more complete construct may be protective for those in high stress and trauma-exposed occupations. This proposal is consistent with the research literature that links mindfulness with emotional stability via an enhanced ability to differentiate and regulate emotion (Hill and Updegraff, 2012).

Based on the mindfulness-resilience relationship, several mindfulness-based interventions are of interest for the purposes of enhancing resilience. In an exploratory study of depressed adults with a history of suicidal ideation or behaviors, MCBT was found to be more effective than treatment as usual at increasing one's meta-awareness and remembering past suicidal ideation in a decentered manner; the absence of these two outcomes often predicts recurrent suicidal ideation and behavior (Hargus, Crane, Barnhofer, and Williams, 2010). Increased mindfulness in vulnerable populations such as found in this study, may enhance resilience when approaching similar thought or behavior patterns in the past that lead to suicidal ideation.

DBT is another mindfulness-based intervention which research studies report promise for individuals coping with past trauma (Iverson, Shenk, and Fruzetti, 2009). Originally developed for people experiencing extreme emotional instability and constant perception of crises, it is logical that it may increase resilience in people high in neuroticism. DBT has been shown to have positive outcomes and promote resiliency in a sample of women that experienced domestic abuse; at post-treatment their depressive symptoms and psychological distress had significantly decreased and their social adjustment had increased (Iverson et al., 2009). Mindfulness-based interventions have even shown promise in promoting resiliency in at-risk youth (Coholic, Eys, and Lougheed, 2012; Semple, Lee, Rosa, Miller, 2010). As a result of the ever increasing literature on mindfulness and its relationships to psychological well-being, predicting that mindfulness may account for the association between neuroticism and resilience is a logical next step in research. Once this model is established, examining mindfulness-based participants of interventions in those higher in neuroticism and measuring resilience outcomes would be an essential addition to the literature.

Mediation and moderation models. The cognitive qualities and emotional outcomes of mindfulness may produce mediation effects on the ineffective attention and awareness that leads to negative reactivity in neuroticism, and provide a stronger relationship with resilience. Three research studies evaluated mediation models that lend support to the idea that mindfulness is a potential mediator of neuroticism (Feltman, et al., 2009; Fetterman et al., 2010; Labbé, et al., 2011).

Feltman, et al. (2009) evaluated the relationships between mindfulness, neuroticism and depressive symptoms in one study and between mindfulness, neuroticism and trait anger in another study with a convenience sample of 289 undergraduate college students. They found that neuroticism was a negative predictor of mindfulness. In addition, both neuroticism and mindfulness were independent predictors for both trait anger and depressive symptoms. They conclude that trait mindfulness functions as a moderator on neuroticism, in that higher levels of mindfulness result in lower levels of anger and depression symptoms.

Fetterman et al. (2010) reported three studies with a convenience sample of 226 undergraduate participants in order to evaluate the role of mindfulness in mediating neuroticism and behavioral dysregulation. Using Baron and Kenny's (1986) procedures they found that mindfulness mediated that effects of neuroticism on behavioral dysregulation. The results of the study indicated that neuroticism was an inverse predictor of mindfulness. Furthermore, higher levels of mindfulness were related to lower levels of impulsivity and higher levels of self-control.

Labbé and colleagues (2011) evaluated resiliency, mindfulness, and psychological and physical health in a convenience sample of 152 college students. Also using Baron and Kenny's (1986) procedures their results indicated that mindfulness was a negative and significant predictor of neuroticism and a positive and significant predictor of resilience. The results also demonstrated that mindfulness partially mediated the effects of neuroticism on resilience.

These initial studies report consistent findings and suggest that mindfulness does have a significant impact on neuroticism, and can increase resilience and decrease negative emotional symptomology. A major limitation of these research studies is they all used a convenience sample of undergraduate students, thus limiting generalization to other populations. Replicating these mediation or moderation models with other populations would provide more information on how these variables relate to a variety of people, particularly with clinical populations.

Conclusion

In summary, neuroticism and resilience appear to be linked in the research literature, but the mechanisms of this relationship remain unclear as it stands in the present literature.

Mindfulness may be an explanatory factor in this association; that is, increased neuroticism is associated with decreased mindfulness, which in turn is associated with decreased resilience. Future research should expand and continue to explore this proposed relationship. If this mediation model stands up to scientific scrutiny, then it may lead us to effective interventions for people that have difficulty coping with life stressors.

Mindfulness-based interventions appear to be an important resource, especially for those individuals that are high in neuroticism. The evidence for the efficacy of mindfulness-based interventions in increasing mindfulness and psychological well-being is strong (e.g., Carmody and Baer, 2008), providing further support for this type of intervention. Additionally, there is some evidence in the research literature that attentional and awareness aspects of mindfulness may account for this relationship (e.g. Giluk, 2009; Bernstein et al., 2011).

Furthermore, the use of the FFMQ (Baer et al., 2006) or other more comprehensive measure of mindfulness may be useful to determine if other factors, such as having a nonjudgmental acceptance in the present moment, decrease neuroticism and promote resilience.

Most facets of mindfulness are traits or cognitive processes that would tend to reduce neuroticism, such that someone who is mindful will not perceive their experience as negative, but will have this radical acceptance without judgment allowing for a more adaptive response.

References

Baer, R. A. (2006). Mindfulness-based treatment approaches: Clinician's guide to evidence base and applications. San Diego, CA US: *Elsevier Academic Press.*

Baer, R. A., Lykins, E. L. B., and Peters, J. R. (2012). Mindfulness and self-compassion as predictors of psychological wellbeing in long-term meditators and matched nonmeditators. *The Journal of Positive Psychology*, *7*, 230-238.

Baer, R. A., Smith, G. T., Hopkins, J., Krietemeyer, J., Toney, L. (2006). Using self-report assessment methods to explore facets of mindfulness. *Assessment, 13*, 27-45.

Barnhofer, T., Duggan, D. S., and Griffith, J. W. (2011). Dispositional mindfulness moderates the relation between neuroticism and depressive symptoms. *Personality And Individual Differences, 51*, 958-962. doi:10.1016/j.paid.2011.07.032.

Baron, R.M., and Kenny, D.A. (1986). The moderator-mediator variable distinction in social psychological research: Conceptual, strategic, and statistical consideration. *Journal of Personality and Social Psychology*, *51*, 1173-1182.

Bernstein, A., Tanay, G., and Vujanovic, A. A. (2011). Concurrent relations between mindful attention and awareness and psychopathology among trauma-exposed adults: Preliminary evidence of transdiagnostic resilience. *Journal of Cognitive Psychotherapy*: *An International Quarterly*, *25*, 99-113.

Block-Lerner, J., Adair, C., Plumb, J. C., Rhatigan, D. L., and Orsillo, S. M. (2007). The case for mindfulness-based approaches in the cultivation of empathy: Does nonjudgmental, present-moment awareness increase capacity for perspective-taking and empathic concern? *Journal of Marital and Family Therapy, 33*, 501-516.

Bonanno, G. A. (2004). Loss, trauma, and human resilience: Have we underestimated the human capacity to thrive after extremely aversive events? *American Psychologist, 59*, 20-28. doi: 10.1037/0003-66X.59.1.20.

Brewin, C. R., Andrews, B., and Valentine, J. D. (2000). Meta-analysis of risk factors for post-traumatic stress disorder in trauma-exposed adults.

Journal of Counseling and Clinical Psychology, 68, 748-766. doi: 10.1037//0022-006X.68.5.748.

Brown, K. W., and Ryan, R. M. (2003). The benefits of being present: Mindfulness and its role in psychological well-being. *Journal of Personality and Social Psychology, 84*, 822-848.

Carmody, J., and Baer, R. A. (2008). Relationships between mindfulness practice and levels of mindfulness, medical and psychological symptoms and well-being in a mindfulness-based stress reduction program. *Journal of Behavioral Medicine, 31*, 23-33.

Coholic, D., Eys, M., and Lougheed, S. (2012). Investigating the effectiveness of an arts-based and mindfulness-based group program for the improvement of resilience in children in need. *Journal of Child and Family Studies, 21*, 833-844.

Costa, P. T., and McCrae, R. R. (1980). Influence of extraversion and neuroticism on subjective well-being: Happy and unhappy people. *Journal Of Personality And Social Psychology, 38*, 668-678. doi:10.1037/0022-3514.38.4.668.

Costa, P. T., McCrae, R. R., and Holland, J. L. (1984). Personality and vocational interests in an adult sample. *Journal Of Applied Psychology, 69*, 390-400. doi:10.1037/0021-9010.69.3.390.

Costa, P. T., and McCrae, R. R. (1992). Revised NEO personality inventory (NEO PI-R) and NEO five-factor inventory (NEO-FFI). Professional manual. Lutz, FL: *Psychological Assessment Resources*.

Dekeyser, M., Raes, F., Leijssen, M., Leysen, S, and Dewulf, D. (2008). Mindfulness skills and interpersonal behavior. *Personality and Individual Differences, 44*, 1235-1245.

Feltman, R., Robinson, M. D., and Ode, S. (2009). Mindfulness as a moderator of neuroticism-outcome relations: A self-regulation perspective. *Journal of Research in Personality, 43*, 953–961.

Fetterman, A. K., Robinson, M. D., Ode, S., and Gordon, K. H. (2010). Neuroticism as a risk factor for behavioral dysregulation: A mindfulness-mediation perspective. *Journal of Social And Clinical Psychology, 29*, 301-321. doi:10.1521/jscp.2010.29.3.301

Friborg, O., Barlaug, D., Martinussen, M., Rosenvinge, J. H., and Hjemdal, O. (2005). Resilience in relation to personality and intelligence. International *Journal of Methods in Psychiatric Research, 14*, 29-42. doi:10.1002/mpr.15

Giluk, T. L. (2009). Mindfulness, Big Five personality, and affect: A meta-analysis. *Personality and Individual Differences*, *47*, 805–811.

Hargus, E., Crane, C., Barnhofer, T., and Williams, J. M. G. (2010). Effects of mindfulness on meta-awareness and specificity in suicidal depression. *Emotion*, *10*, 34-42.

Hill, C. L. M., and Updegraff, J. A. (2012). Mindfulness and its relationship to emotional regulation. *Emotion, 12*, 81-90.

Hjemdal, O., Friborg, O., Martinussen, M., and Rosenvinge, J.H. (2001). Preliminary results from the development and validation of a Norwegian scale for measuring adult resilience. *Journal of Norwegian Psychology Association 38*, 310-17.

Hofmann, S. G., Sawyer, A. T., Witt, A. A., and Oh, D. (2010). The effect of mindfulness-based therapy on anxiety and depression: A meta-analytic review. *Journal of Consulting and Clinical Psychology, 78*, 169–183.

Iverson, K. M., Shenk, C., and Fruzzetti, A. E. (2009). Dialectical behavior therapy for women victims of domestic abuse: A pilot study. *Professional Psychology: Research and Practice*, *40*, 242-248.

Jacobs, T. L., Epel, E. S., Lin, J., Blackburn, E.H., Wolkowitz, O. M., Bridwell, D.A., Zanesco, A. P., Aichele, S. R., Sahdra, B. K., MacLean, K. A., King, B. G., Shaver, P. R., Rosenberg, E. L., Ferrer, E., Wallace, B. A., and Saron, C. D. (2011). Intensive meditation trainng, immune cell, telomerase activity, and psychological mediators. *Psychoneuro-endocrinology, 36*, 664-681.

Kabat-Zinn, J. (1990). *Full Catastrophe Living: Using the Wisdom of Your Body and Mind to Face Stress, Pain, and Illness*. New York, NY: Bantam Dell.

Keng, S. L., Smoski, M. J., and Robins, C. J. (2011). Effects of mindfulness on psychological health: A review of empirical studies. *Clinical Psychology Review, 31*, 1041-1056.

Labbé, E. (2011). *Psychology Moment by Moment: A Guide to Enhancing Your Clinical Practice with Mindfulness and Meditation*. Oakland, CA: New Harbinger Publications.

Labbé, E. E., Womble, M., Shenesey, J. (2011). Exploring the relationship between mindfulness and resilience. In Stark, C.A. and Bonner, D.C. (Eds.), *Handbook on Spirituality: Belief Systems, Societal Impact and Roles in Coping*. Hauppauge, NY: Nova Science Publishers, Inc.

Labbé, E. E., Womble, M., Shenesey, J., Chavers, D., Wilson, K., (2012). Evaluation of the Psychometric Properties of the Resilience Questionnaire. In Submission.

Lent, J., and Schwartz, R. C. (2012). The impact of work setting, demographic characteristics, and personality factors related to burnout among professional counselors. *Journal Of Mental Health Counseling*, *34*, 355-372.

McCrae, R. R., (1999). Mainstream Personality Psychology and the Study of Religion. *Journal of Personality*, *67*, 1209-1218.

Neenan, M. (2009*). Developing resilience: A Cognitive-Behavioral Approach*. New York, New York: Routledge.

Pargament, K. I. (1997). *The psychology of religion and coping: Theory, research, practice*. New York: Guilford.

Pargament, K. I., and Brant, C. R., (1998). Religion and Coping. In Koenig, H. G. (Ed.), *Handbook of Religion and Mental Health*. San Diego: Academic Press.

Semple, R. J., Lee, J., Rosa, D., and Miller, L. F. (2010). A randomized trial of mindfulness-based cognitive therapy for children: Promoting mindful attention to enhance social-emotional resiliency in children. *Journal of Child and Family Studies, 19*, 218-229.

Sideroff, S. I., (2004). Resilience: A Functional Approach to Stress. California Biofeedback, 20.

Smith, B. W., Ortiz, J. A., Steffen, L. E., Tooley, E. M., Wiggins, K. T., Yeater, E. A., Montoya, J. D., and Bernard, M. L. (2011). Mindfulness is associated with few PTSD symptoms, depressive symptoms, physical symptoms, and alcohol problems in urban firefighters. *Journal of Counseling and Clinical Psychology*, *79*, 613-617.

Van den Hurk, P. A. M., Wingens, T., Giommi, F., Barendregt, H. P., Speckens, A. E. M., and van Schie, H. T. (2011). On the relationship between the practice of mindfulness meditation and personality—an exploratory analysis of the mediating role of mindfulness skills. *Mindfulness, 2*, 194-200.

Wachs, K., and Cordova, J. V. (2007). Mindful relating: Exploring mindfulness and emotion repertoires in intimate relationships. *Journal of Marital and Family Therapy*, *33*, 464-481.

Wagnild, G. M. and Young, H. M. (1993). Development and psychometric evaluation of the Resilience Scale. *Journal of Nursing Measurement,* 1, 165-178.

Williams, V., Ciarrochi, J., and Deane, F. P. (2010). On being mindful, emotionally aware, and more resilient: Longitudinal pilot study of police recruits. *Australian Psychologist*, *45*, 274-282.

INDEX

E

F

G

H

I

J

K

L

M

T

U

V